# Does the United States Need a National Health Insurance Policy?

# Does the United States Need a National Health Insurance Policy?

Other books in the At Issue series:

# At ✳ Issue

# Does the United States Need a National Health Insurance Policy?

Nancy Harris, *Book Editor*

Bruce Glassman, *Vice President*
Bonnie Szumski, *Publisher*
Helen Cothran, *Managing Editor*

**GREENHAVEN PRESS**
*An imprint of Thomson Gale, a part of The Thomson Corporation*

34000200028025

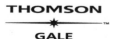

THOMSON
GALE

Detroit • New York • San Francisco • San Diego • New Haven, Conn.
Waterville, Maine • London • Munich

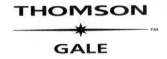

LIBRARY OF CONGRESS CATALOGING-IN-PUBLICATION DATA

Does the United States need a national health insurance policy? / Nancy Harris, book editor.
    p. cm. — (At issue)
Includes bibliographical references and index.
ISBN 0-7377-3188-5 (lib. : alk. paper) — ISBN 0-7377-3189-3 (pbk. : alk. paper)
    1. National health insurance—United States. I. Harris, Nancy, 1952– . II. At issue (San Diego, Calif.)
RA412.2.D64 2006
368.4'2'00973—dc22                                                            2005040273

Printed in the United States of America

# Contents

# Introduction

Health care reform has been a contentious issue for many years in the United States. Most Americans agree that the current system is not working. According to Harvard economist David M. Cutler, "The problems of medical care confront us daily. . . . Barely one in five Americans thinks the medical system works well." Those concerned with improving the system often look to other nations for reform models. All industrialized nations except for the United States have some sort of universal health care system. Within these universal health care systems there are major differences, including the way nations fund their health care, how the health care is delivered, and the role the government plays in each system.

In the United States, health care is primarily paid for with private insurance and is predominantly managed by health maintenance organizations (HMOs). HMOs are organizations that offer health insurance and are part of "managed care" plans. These plans were implemented in the United States in the early 1990s to help control national health care costs, which had been rising steadily. HMOs offer lower premiums (insurance payments) than most traditional health plans. With an HMO plan, a patient must choose a primary care physician from the HMO's network of doctors and must get this doctor's approval for all exams, hospital visits, and referrals to medical specialists. By limiting patients' access to expensive specialists and procedures, HMOs aim to reduce costs.

Although supporters argue that HMOs have saved the United States billions of dollars in health care spending, critics charge that in order to cut costs, HMOs have limited access to vital services because they have operated primarily for their own profit. Moreover, insurance rates have escalated, leaving many Americans unable to afford health care coverage. For those who cannot afford health insurance, the government has public insurance plans, including Medicaid and Medicare, for the poor, the elderly, and veterans. Nevertheless, an estimated 40 million Americans remain uninsured. In addition, many American workers have health insurance plans that provide very poor coverage. As stated by political scientists Kant Patel and Mark E. Rushefsky, "Private insurance . . . leaves a portion of the population underinsured and vulnerable to catastrophic medical expenses." To remedy these problems, reformers have looked to the universal health care systems of other nations.

There are basically two types of universal health care systems: One is mostly public, and the other is a mix of public and private. In the first, health care is paid for through general taxation or payroll taxes. Publicly owned hospitals employing salaried doctors provide health care in what is commonly called socialized medicine. Sweden, Italy, and Great Britain have variations of this type of socialized medicine. Great Britain's health care system, for example, is funded and administered by the national government's National Health Service (NHS). The NHS owns and operates over two thousand hospitals and directly employs most hospital staff and most physicians. British citizens are not obligated to participate in the NHS, and about 11 percent of the British population chooses to be insured privately. In the British health care system, citizens have access to a primary care physician, with some limitations on whom they may see at no charge, and obtain prescription drugs for less than four dollars per prescription. There are no hospital or physician charges for tests or in-hospital treatment.

In more mixed systems, health care is mostly publicly financed through payroll taxes, but private hospitals and doctors deliver the health care services. Germany, Japan, France, Holland, and Canada have such hybrid systems.

Many Americans who are concerned about U.S. health care advocate adopting a system similar to Canada's. Basically, Canadians have a Medicare-style plan for their entire country. However, private insurance still exists in Canada for services not covered by the plan, such as dental care and the cost of some prescription medications. Like other universal health care systems, Canada dispenses care on the basis of need, not individual finances. As a result, all Canadians have access to necessary medical services, which must be provided regardless of age, prior condition, location, or employment. In addition, because Canada has a simple billing system, health care administrative costs are drastically lower than in the United States, where hospitals and physicians must deal with thousands of insurance companies.

Canada's health care system may seem like an appealing alternative; however, implementing Canada's (or any other nation's) system in the United States would generate far-reaching changes such as possible tax increases and the breakup of private health insurance companies nationwide. Although many critics of adopting a health care system like Canada's are concerned about the changes that would necessarily accompany such a drastic restructuring, many are more concerned with the basic nature of universal health care. Many Americans believe that publicly funded health care is a form of socialism. These critics argue that America's free market can deliver health care more efficiently than can the government.

Modeling America's health care system after another nation's would obviously create many challenges. The authors in *At Issue: Does the United States Need a National Health Insurance Policy?* give numerous perspectives on how to reform the U.S. health care system. As this anthology makes clear, the question of whether to adopt a national health insurance policy generates intense debate.

# 1

# The United States Needs a National Health Insurance Policy

## Donald L. Barlett and James B. Steele

*Donald L. Barlett and James B. Steele are investigative jour-
nalists who have worked as a team for thirty years. They
have worked for the* Philadelphia Inquirer *and as editors at
large for* Time *magazine. They also have won two Pulitzer
Prizes and two National Magazine Awards. Barlett and
Steele are coauthors of six books, including* America: What
Went Wrong?, The Great American Tax Dodge, *and*
America: Who Stole the Dream?

America's health care system comprises a fragmented
collection of businesses, government agencies, health
care facilities, and educational institutions. In addition,
thousands of special interest groups such as the American Cancer Society wage campaigns to shape American
health care policy with no regard for what is best for
American health care overall. The best remedy would
be to implement a national single-payer system that
would have one agency to collect all medical fees and
pay all claims. This system would eliminate the bureaucratic waste created by thousands of individual health
plans. Moreover, under a single-payer plan, all Americans would receive basic comprehensive health care as
well as have the freedom to choose their own doctor
and hospital, choices that are missing in the present
market-driven health care model.

Donald L. Bartlett and James B. Steele, *Critical Condition: How Health Care in
America Became Big Business and Bad Medicine.* New York: Doubleday, 2004. Copyright © 2004 by Donald L. Barlett and James B. Steele. Reproduced by permission
of Doubleday, a division of Random House, Inc.

The D-Day invasion of June 6, 1944, which would turn the tide of World War II for the Allies, was the largest amphibious assault in the history of warfare. Altogether, 5,000 ships, 13,000 aircraft, and 180,000 men took part in the initial landing on the coast of France. While not everything went according to plan, D-Day was both an incredible military success and a spectacular triumph of organization.

But imagine what would have happened if the American, British, and Canadian military units each had gone its own way instead of following a coordinated master plan. Suppose that each of the U.S. Army's twenty divisions had assembled its own list of targets, with the 101st Airborne Division dropping into one part of France, the 82nd Airborne into another. Suppose that each company within each of those divisions had done likewise. Then imagine the same for the British and Canadians: 180,000 troops, each man marching to his own drummer.

## No System at All

That is precisely the picture of the U.S. health care system today, thousands of individual entities heading off in many directions on missions that frequently conflict. It's really no system at all. Rather, it's a stunningly fragmented collection of businesses, government agencies, health care facilities, educational institutions, and other special interests wasting tens of billions of dollars and turning the treatment of disease and sickness into a lottery where some losers pay with their lives.

> *The simplest and most cost-effective remedy would be to provide universal coverage and to create one agency to collect medical fees and pay claims.*

The United States has 6,000 hospitals and tens of thousands more freestanding medical centers, nursing homes, kidney dialysis centers, laboratories, MRI facilities, pharmacies, and medical schools. Each maintains its own computer system. Some can talk to one another; most can't. Overlying these are hundreds of HMOs, private insurers, and government plans. There's Medicaid for the very poor, Medicare for everyone over sixty-five years of age, TRICARE and the Veterans Administration for the military, and a hodgepodge for everyone else. Each insurer has its own system of co-pays, deductibles, and spending limits. Each produces thousands of pages of impenetrable language setting forth the medical expenses it will pay, the ones it won't, and those that fall somewhere in between.

> *To discredit the single-payer idea, insurers, HMOS, for-profit hospitals, and other private interests play on Americans' long-standing fears of big government.*

Then there are thousands of special interests, from the American Cancer Society to the American Medical Association, from the Pharmaceutical Research and Manufacturers of America (PhRMA) to the American Organ Transplant Association, each with its own agenda. Each wages an individual campaign to shape health care policy by manipulating public opinion through TV, newspapers, magazines, and radio. Each seeks to grab a piece of the health care pie. Out of all these thousands of self-interested entities, not one speaks for what's best for American health care overall.

## U.S. Health Care Is Second-Rate

And that explains why U.S. health care is second-rate at the start of the twenty-first century and destined to get a lot worse and much more expensive. It's why some people must hold garage sales to pay their medical bills, why almost no one knows what their health insurance will pay for until it's too late. It's why many Americans are forced to make job choices based not on what they might like to do in life, or what's in their best interest, but on the health insurance packages offered by employers. It's why U.S. corporations are at a disadvantage in a global economy, forced to divert ever more revenue and resources to administering health care plans. It's why some diseases such as colon cancer or attention deficit disorder, which capture the media's attention, get a substantial share of government research and treatment dollars, while other diseases that receive less attention, such as amyotrophic lateral sclerosis (Lou Gehrig's disease) and cystic fibrosis, receive far fewer dollars. It's why millions of Americans are forced to agonize over how to care for aging parents with Alzheimer's disease, or how to pay the bills for children with a catastrophic illness—and do so without depriving siblings of their needs. It's why millions of Americans needlessly consume expensive medications that enrich pharmaceutical companies and Wall Street, but that contribute little or nothing to a longer, healthier life. Finally, it explains why Americans are the most overtreated, undertreated, and mistreated health care patients on earth.

It need not be this way.

## Provide Universal Coverage

The simplest and most cost-effective remedy would be to provide universal coverage and to create one agency to collect medical fees and pay claims. This would eliminate the staggering overlap, duplication, bureaucracy, and waste created by thousands of individual plans, the hidden costs that continue to drive health care out of reach for a steadily growing number of Americans.

Under a single-payer system, all health care providers—doctors, hospitals, clinics—would bill one agency for their services and would be reimbursed by the same agency. Every American would receive basic comprehensive health care, including essential prescription drugs and rehabilitative care. Anyone who needed to be treated or hospitalized could receive medical care without having to wrestle with referrals and without fear of financial ruin. Complex billing procedures and ambiguities over what is covered by insurance would be eliminated.

> *What's needed is a fresh approach, a new organization that is independent and free from politics.*

Radical? We already have universal health care and a single-payer system for everybody aged sixty-five and over: It's called Medicare. For years, researchers, think tanks, citizens' groups, and health care professionals have advocated a similar plan for the rest of the population. Study after study has concluded that the most practical and cost-effective way to provide quality health care and to restrain costs is a single-payer system, but no plan has ever come close to adoption because of fierce opposition by the powerful health care lobby.

To discredit the single-payer idea, insurers, HMOs, for-profit hospitals, and other private interests play on Americans' long-standing fears of big government. This view was summed up by Susan Pisano, a vice president of the American Association of Health Plans, who contended in 2002 that a single-payer system "would lead to the creation of a large federal bureaucracy that would be less responsive and actually raise issues of cost, access and quality more than it would solve them."

## The Private Market Has Created a Massive Bureaucracy

In truth, it is the private market that has created a massive bureaucracy, one that dwarfs the size and costs of Medicare, the most efficiently run health insurance program in America in terms of administrative costs. Medicare's overhead averages about 2 percent a year. In a 2002 study for Maine, Mathematica Policy Research Inc. concluded that administrative costs of private insurers in the state ranged from 12 percent to more than 30 percent. Studies of private carriers in other areas have reached similar conclusions. This isn't surprising, because unlike Medicare, which relies on economies of scale and standardized universal coverage, private insurance is built on bewilderingly complex layers of plans and providers that require a costly bureaucracy to administer, much of which is geared toward denying claims.

Some studies have put the price tag for administering the current system at nearly one out of every three health care dollars, much higher than that of any nation with single-payer health care. There is no way of knowing how much the United States could save by adopting such a system, but even with one that covered 100 percent of the population, the savings would be substantial.

What kind of an agency would administer it?

## Create a New Agency

The idea of a single-payer plan run by the U.S. government carries with it far too much political baggage ever to get off the ground. What's needed is a fresh approach, a new organization that is independent and free from politics, one that can focus with laserlike precision on what needs to be done to further the health interests of everyone in a fair manner. For in addition to covering the basic costs of all Americans, a new system needs to institute programs that will improve America's overall health, that will focus on preventing illness and disease as well as treatment, and do so without breaking the bank.

How does the United States come up with such a mechanism?

One possible answer: Loosely copy and then amend and expand on what already exists in another setting—the Federal Reserve System, a quasigovernmental organization that oversees the nation's money and banking policies. The Fed is one of the nation's most ingenious creations, a public agency that is largely independent of politics. The Fed's board members are appointed to staggered fourteen-year terms by the President with the consent of the Senate, meaning that neither the White House nor Congress can substantively influence the Fed's policies.

## The U.S. Council on Health Care

Call this independent agency the U.S. Council on Health Care (USCHC). Like the Federal Reserve, the council would set an overall policy for health care and influence its direction by controlling federal spending—from managing research grants to providing basic and catastrophic medical coverage for all citizens. Unlike the Federal Reserve, it would be entirely funded by taxpayers. The money could come from just two taxes, a gross-receipts levy on businesses and a flat tax, similar to the current Medicare tax, on all individual income, not just wages. This would not represent an additional cost to society, but rather replace existing taxes and write-offs. It would cut costs for corporations and raise taxes slightly on individuals at the top of the income ladder. Members of the USCHC board would include both health care professionals and citizens from all walks of life. Its mission: Implement policies that improve health care for everyone, not just those suffering from certain diseases. In short, make the unpopular decisions that the market cannot make.

The council could establish regions similar to those of the Federal Reserve System, which divides the nation into twelve areas. Whatever their number, the geographic subdivisions could take into account cultural and regional differences among Americans. They would allow for health care delivery to be fine-tuned at the local level, and ensure that regulations could take into account the differences between metropolitan and community hospitals.

Although the USCHC could be set up to keep partisan politics out of hospitals and doctors' offices, health care politics, which can be every bit as divisive as the mainstream variety, would still present a challenge. If you have any doubt, just assemble surgeons, radiologists, and internists in a room to discuss the merits of their particular approaches to treatment of a specific disease. But those members of a USCHC board drawn from outside the health care community would at least introduce a moderating influence.

# 2

# The United States Does Not Need a National Health Insurance Policy

## David C. MacDonald

*David C. MacDonald is a practicing physician in Renton, Washington. He is a founder of the American Association of Patients and Providers, a nonprofit organization aimed at finding solutions to health care problems that do not burden the taxpayer. MacDonald is also a national speaker for the American Osteopathic Association and other physicians' organizations.*

In a national single-payer health care system, every individual's health care would be paid for by one federal agency, which would allow too much government control over health care choices. Single-payer systems have not worked well anywhere else in the world, and Americans should not expect that they would work in the United States. In lieu of a single-payer system, alternative programs could provide solutions by helping the uninsured pay for their health care through community volunteer work.

Imagine this scenario: You just purchased a new car. The salesperson explains that all new-car owners must participate in a new program: "Managed Car." This is an attempt to cut down on the paperwork and waste associated with the operation of an automobile. Your service representative will help you locate the "best" (cheapest) oil to buy and the "best" (cheapest) service locations participating in their program and will help you avoid costly, preventive maintenance. They also will help you avoid those who might take advantage of you by recommending wasteful additives or synthetic oils that are more expensive and outside the mainstream of auto maintenance.

## How a Single-Payer System Might Function

Sound ridiculous? I agree, but the above is a close parallel to what would happen under a single-payer health-insurance program. Imagine another scenario: You walk into the grocery store and there is a sign at the entrance stating that there is a new program for the county, the "County Single-Payer Food Program," for all county residents. After all, food is a right and our country should not let anyone starve to death. Food prices no longer would be posted, for fear that the store managers might compromise their commitment to their customers. So you meander through the store and you enjoy purchasing without regard for the cost of the products. In fact, it is not long before your food selections change from previous trips to the same store. The T-bone steaks seem more attractive, the lobster finds its way into your basket and you pass by the day-old bread section you used to frequent. As you enter the check-out line the cashier presents you with the total bill: $110.89. You present your Single-Payer Food Group card, the cashier makes a note on the receipt and you leave the store. Six months later, the Single-Payer County Food Group writes to you stating they mailed a check to the grocery store for $37.65, the usual and customary amount for the food you purchased.

> *The stark reality is a single-payer system has not worked well anywhere in the world.*

These scenarios are not far from the reality of what managed-care organizations have done to our health-care system and how a single-payer system may function. Our society never would let the government determine where our car should be serviced, the type of gasoline we may buy and how often we are able to change the oil in our car. Why do we let this happen with our health care?

What is so attractive about a single-payer system? For the patients, there is the perception that whenever they are ill, a medical facility will be waiting with open arms to take care of them. For the physicians, there is the lure of less paperwork and the freedom to practice their art without the complexities associated with billing. For the politicians, health-care decisions attract voters who are hopeful that somehow the central government will be able to stabilize the fear of our ailing health-care system. Many who are not familiar with the actual health-care delivery system in other countries often cite partial truths that imply the grass is greener in a single-payer environment. Many use Canada as a country for the United States to emulate, without knowing how their system functions. Last Jan. 2 [1999] 23 of the 25 hospital emergency rooms in Toronto were closed to patients, regardless of the severity of their illness. Canada has long waiting lists for medical technology such as MRI [magnetic resonance imaging] and CT [computerized tomography] scanners. According to the Vancouver-based Fraser Institute, studies show that in 1997–98 about 170,000 people in British Columbia were not covered because they had not paid premiums required by the province. Alberta also requires a premium and does not cover individuals who do not pay. A 1999 poll found that 76 percent of Canadians now believe the health-care system is in crisis.

## Many Uninsured Choose Not to Have Insurance

Those who favor a central-government single-payer system often cite the millions who are uninsured as the main reason for the need for universal coverage. However, the number of uninsured is a very soft number. According to the U.S. Census Bureau, in 1998 3.5 million of the uninsured had incomes that exceeded $75,000/year. According to a 1996 survey, 6.3 million had access to health insurance and chose not to pay for it. Actually, medical costs are low for most of us, according to the *Journal of American Health Policy*. They report that 33 percent of the U.S. population have no medical expenses each year. Another 40 percent spend less than $500 per year and only 3 percent spend more than $5,000 per year. A question we must consider is: Are we paying inflated fees for insurance that is not paying for what Americans are asking for?

The stark reality is a single-payer system has not worked well anywhere in the world. Why do some Americans believe we can make it work here? As a practicing family physician, it is frustrating to listen to theoretical arguments for a single-payer system. A far different reality belies the theory, such as the university hospital in the Southwest that advertised for much of the local surgical business. Not long after a successful advertising campaign, they realized that they could not perform the procedures for the price they advertised.

## Single-Payer Systems Are Similar to Managed Care

Ironically, managed-care systems function much like a single-payer program because decisions are made at a distance from the consumer. A study by Deloitte and Touche, a consulting firm, found that consumers are not satisfied with managed care. Sixty-two percent believe HMOs make it harder to see specialists; 61 percent believe they have less time with their patients in an HMO environment; and 43 percent are not satisfied with access to their physician. According to the *Yankelovich Monitor* [a publication that studies consumer trends], 70 percent of physicians surveyed characterized themselves as against managed care; 46 percent often think about leaving clinical practice; and the hassle factor has increased due to restrictions on the ability to treat, cumbersome preauthorization and prolonged reimbursement time. California certainly has had challenges with health care. According to Price Waterhouse [a business that provides advice to public and private clients] health-care premiums continue to increase despite declining payments to the physicians. Patients, physicians and politicians are so frustrated that many are ready to accept anything that may provide relief.

> *We should allow the free market to establish the 'true' insurance costs by removing the mandated benefits.*

Most patients and providers are unaware of the actual costs for clinic visits, hospitalizations, procedures and medications. As a result, the utilization rate for services usually is distorted. Some services may be underutilized, such as preventive care, or others may be overutilized, such as emergency rooms. Studies have found that if the patient participation is high enough (with additional charges for after-hour services), the utilization rate declines. Some of the positive aspects that have surfaced as a result of managed care are the waste and inflated fees for some services. Physicians, hospitals, vendors, research projects, patients and pharmaceutical companies are all responsible for our inflated health-care costs.

Major medical policies are affordable very similar to high-deductible car insurance. If we had insurance to cover our gasoline, tires and wiper blades, our car insurance would be outrageous. In essence, health insurance is so expensive because we are trying to insure services and products that should not fall under the insurance umbrella. Small-business owners constantly are trying to find a reasonable health-insurance program for their employees. As a result, some employees change health plans yearly. Continuity of care is lost, patient choice is almost unheard of and premiums continue to increase while satisfaction wanes.

Another reality is that costs have increased in all aspects of society. A recent visit by my plumber reminded me that outpatient health-care costs are no more expensive than other services provided. The fear of the major medical events is what drives us all to purchase health insurance.

## Patients Should Determine Their Health Care

However, there is a single-payer system that requires no legislation to implement, already has demonstrated its ability to control costs, empowers patient choice, maintains individual privacy and increases access to care. Who is the single payer in this system? The patient! Patients are the best ones to determine the type of health care they should receive. If patients have the incentive to remain well, and if they have access to unspent health-care dollars, they will make very wise health-care decisions.

My partner, Dr. Vern Cherewatenko, and I started a non-profit group, the American Association of Patients and Providers, to develop solutions to our health-care dilemma that are not a burden to the taxpayers. One program, SimpleCare, eliminates the administrative waste and passes the savings back to the patient. This program initially was developed to help the uninsured. However, the program is also a boon to consumers who have a major medical policy and would like to retain the decision-making authority regarding their health-care dollars. Patients are able to decide the integrative-medicine aspects that meet their needs without the hassle of preauthorization. Patients and providers are thrilled with this program.

Another nonprofit program developed for the uninsured or those who are unable to pay is Cares for America. Patients are seen and a charge generated similar to SimpleCare. The patient then has 90 days to volunteer his or her time with participating community programs. Takin' It to the Streets is a similar program. Providers bring health care to a needy part of the community in exchange for work, such as sweeping the streets, picking up trash or planting flowers.

As employers continue to get out of the health-care industry, there are fewer options for individuals. We should allow the free market to establish the "true" insurance costs by removing the mandated benefits. We also should remove the barrier for medical-savings accounts and allow patients to determine where their health-care dollars are spent.

# 3

# A National Health Insurance Policy Would Be Superior to Market-Based Plans

## Kip Sullivan

*Kip Sullivan is a member of the steering committee of the Health Care Campaign of Minnesota. He has worked as an attorney organizing Minnesota's Citizens Organized Acting Together, a statewide citizen group founded in the 1970s. While working for COACT, he coordinated a universal coverage campaign and worked on health policy. He has written about health policy for newspapers, magazines, and journals, including the* New York Times, *the* Los Angeles Times, *the* New England Journal of Medicine, *the* Nation, *and the* Washington Monthly.

Those interested in health care reform have proposed three solutions to remedy the problems associated with managed care: managed competition, large deductibles, and a single-payer system. Managed competition and large deductibles are market-based proposals. Proponents of managed competition believe that greedy doctors prescribe unnecessary drugs and treatments in order to increase their share of the insurance money paid to cover the costs of the medicines and procedures. By utilizing managed care to limit what doctors each patient can see, insurance companies gain more control over the doctors in their group and can thereby cut costs. Advocates of large-deductible plans are hostile to-

Kip Sullivan, "Understanding Health Care Reform Debate: A Primer for the Perplexed," *Social Policy*, vol. 33, Winter 2002–2003. Copyright © 2002 by Kip Sullivan. Reproduced by permission.

ward these managed care plans. They claim that allowing patients to opt for high deductibles in order to cut premiums provides them with a way to reduce their own health care costs. Advocates of a single-payer system, which replaces numerous insurers with one payer, believe that competition and large deductible plans have never worked to solve health care problems. They say that managed care has not driven down health care costs, and high deductibles hurt the chronically ill, who have to pay more out-of-pocket costs than they would have with lower-deductible plans.

Most of us need to help defining the problem. We are all too familiar with it. Our health care system is obscenely expensive, 15 percent of us are uninsured, and about twice that number are underinsured (the underinsured have insurance with big holes that leave them exposed to bankrupting medical bills). Moreover, the spread of managed care has damaged the quality of health care and destroyed patient privacy.

## Three Types of Solutions

Articulating a solution to this mess is more difficult. For the last three decades, three types of solutions have been put forward—managed competition (which relies on "competition" between HMOs), large deductibles, and a single-payer system (a system in which one payer reimburses doctors and hospitals and other "providers"). The first two proposals—managed competition and large deductibles—are market-based proposals. They rest on the assumption that competition can be made to work in the health care sector. Advocates of a single-payer system, on the other hand, believe competition has never worked well, and in some parts of the health care industry it doesn't work at all.

> *Today, the only thing that distinguishes HMOs from non-HMOs is that HMOs limit choice of primary care doctor[s].*

Advocates of managed competition and large deductibles share the belief that "overuse" of medical care explains the high cost of health care in the US. The difference between the two schools is that managed competition advocates believe overuse is caused by greedy doctors, while large-deductible buffs blame "over-insured" patients. Single-payer advocates, on the other hand, blame waste in the system—for example, excessive administrative costs and outrageous drug prices.

## Managed Competition

The phrase "managed competition" was not used until the mid-1980s (it was apparently invented by Alain Enthoven, a Stanford economist). But the cornerstone of managed competition —HMOs—was laid in 1973 when Congress passed the Health Maintenance Organization (HMO) Act. That law subsidized the formation of HMOs, and required employers with 50 or more employees to offer HMOs to their employees if an HMO was operating in the employer's market. HMOs pioneered the cost-control tactics that, by the 1980s, were collectively referred to as "managed care." Managed care refers to financial incentives to doctors to deny care to patients, and to "utilization review" [when HMOs review and decide what treatment patients can receive], which means an HMO employee second-guesses decisions made by doctors and patients.

Thanks to the 1973 HMO Act, the HMO industry grew. Because HMOs had the tools to force doctors to deny services, they had an advantage over traditional insurers (like Blue Cross/Blue Shield and Prudential) which allowed HMOs to keep their premiums five to ten percent below those of the traditional insurers. In the 1980s, as the traditional insurers began to lose market share to the HMOs, they began to adopt managed care tactics. Today, the only thing that distinguishes HMOs from non-HMOs is that HMOs limit choice of primary care doctor. Virtually all non-HMO insurers today use financial incentives and/or some form of utilization review. The traditional insurance company is virtually extinct.

According to health policy experts, only managed care insurers which limit your choice of primary care doctor are HMOs. (HMOs limit choice in order to be able to funnel more patients to the doctors in their network and thereby increase their leverage over the doctors they do select. If an HMO controls 50 percent of a clinic's patients, it has a lot more clout over the doctors who practice in that clinic than it does if it controls only 5 percent of the clinic's patients.) But the public and most reporters use the term HMO to describe any insurer that uses managed care tactics. The HMO that Helen Hunt swore at in the movie *As Good as it Gets* may or may not have been an HMO; it might have been a Blue Cross company using utilization review to deny her asthmatic son the tests he needed. I will use "HMO" from here on as the public uses the term.

## Reforms to Increase Competition

Although HMOs were widespread by the mid-1980s, health care inflation became torrid in the latter half of the 1980s. In 1989, Alain Enthoven and Richard Kronick published a two-part paper in the *New England Journal of Medicine* in which they argued that HMOs should not be blamed for their inability to tame inflation. They said competition between HMOs and traditional insurers wasn't strong enough, and that to make competition more rigorous, it would have to be "managed." They recommended three reforms, all focusing on the demand side, or the buyer's side, of the market.

> *Unfortunately, patient protection laws, with the exception of the right to sue HMOs, are of little value.*

First, they argued that consumers and most employers are too small to force the big insurers to bargain with them over premiums. The solution to this problem was to have consumers join large purchasing coalitions (Enthoven and Kronick called them "sponsors"). Second, they made the dubious assumption that employers and consumers weren't sufficiently angry about the cost of health insurance. To fix this non-problem, they proposed eliminating the tax incentives that lower the effective cost of premiums for both employers and employees. This would make consumers more "cost-conscious," they said. Third, Enthoven and Kronick recommended that someone produce "report cards" on each of the nation's 1,000-plus insurance companies so that sponsors and individual consumers could know which insurer had better quality of care. They didn't indicate who would create sponsors and publish report cards. They simply called for sponsors and report cards, plus a repeal of the tax breaks, and claimed these changes would turn consumers into powerful, cost-conscious, informed buyers, and this in turn would provoke real competition between the HMOs.

By 1989, I had been studying health policy for only three years, but even I could tell that managed competition resembled theology more than economics. The theory suffered numerous problems. I focus here on just two unfixable defects—the high administrative costs of HMOs and their providers, and the negative influence of HMOs on quality of care.

## Costs Increase with HMOs

Administrative costs are those that are not expenditures on health care for patients. Both insurers and providers generate administrative costs. In the insurer sector, administrative costs include expenditures on marketing, underwriting (which refers to the process of doing research on the health histories of applicants to see if the insurance company should insure them and, if so, at what premium level), utilization review, and lobbying, as well as profit. In the provider sector, administrative costs include expenditures on clinic and hospital staff who have to argue with HMO employees about utilization review and about getting paid.

Both anecdotal and empirical evidence indicate administrative costs soared as managed care spread. Between 1968 and 1993, the period in which HMOs took over the system, the number of full-time administrative employees in both the insurer and provider sectors grew 288 percent compared to 159 percent for all medical personnel and a mere 77 percent for physicians. These figures and other data indicate that the savings HMOs achieved by denying medical services to patients were offset by increased administrative costs.

## Report Cards Don't Work

The other unfixable flaw in managed competition was the infeasibility of plan report cards. Report cards on a single service performed by a single doctor or a team of health care professionals, such as bypass surgery, are feasible and in fact have been published in a few states. But report cards on entire HMOs are not. HMOs, like traditional insurance companies, insure for the great majority of the 7,000-plus services for which doctors bill these days. Can you imagine the cost of preparing "grades," every year, on the quality not only of by-pass surgery, but bunionectomy, stroke rehabilitation, mammography, and thousands of other medical services? Can you imagine doing that for each of the nation's 1,000-plus HMOs and other insurers? Can you imagine wading through these behemoth documents and figuring out which HMO is the best?

> *We are, in short, drifting toward the worst of all possible worlds—a world in which managed care policies with large deductibles dominate the market.*

In any event, useful plan report cards never appeared, consumers were never able to put upward pressure on quality to counteract the downward pressure of HMOs, and, surprise, surprise, quality deteriorated as HMOs spread. Polls indicate quality deteriorated, and so does scientific research. The damage to quality became so widespread during the mid-nineties that an "HMO backlash" became visible in 1996. That year, Congress and a majority of state legislatures began debating "patient protection" legislation. Unfortunately, patient protection laws, with the exception of the right to sue HMOs, are of little value. Unless we are prepared to place cops in every examining room, there's little society can do to stop HMOs from damaging quality of care. There are just too many ways for HMOs to short-change patients, and patients, especially those who never went to medical school and who are sick, are poorly equipped to detect and resist HMO rationing and corner-cutting.

## Large-Deductible Policies

The business community tolerated the HMO backlash, but it had little patience with the return of torrid premium inflation. Premium inflation was low from about 1992 to 1996, thanks not to HMO "efficiency" but, rather, to a huge drop in the economy-wide inflation rate and to the merger madness that struck the entire health care industry in 1993. But premium inflation returned with a vengeance in the late 1990s, and hit double-digits in 2000 even though the underlying inflation rate remained unusually low. By then, the business community, which ten years earlier had hailed HMOs as its savior, was entertaining yet another faddish health policy.

The new fad goes by several labels, the most common of which are "defined-contribution plans" and "consumer-driven policies." These phrases refer to health insurance policies with gigantic deductibles, typically in the range of $3,000 to $4,000 for family coverage and $1,000 to $2,000 for individual coverage. The incentive to buy these policies, for both employer and employee, is reduced premiums. (These days, employees are paying 20 to 30 percent of premiums, a percent which may rise sharply in the near future).

Employers who purchase these policies give employees a chunk of money—say, $2,000 to someone buying family coverage—which employees use to pay toward their medical bills. If employees incur medical bills over $2,000, they pay for those bills out of their own pockets until they meet their deductible (say, $4,000), at which point the insurance company begins paying. The great majority of healthy employees with healthy dependents—perhaps 75 percent of all Americans—won't spend $2,000 a year on doctors, hospitals and drugs. For these people, defined-contribution policies promise lower premiums with what are, effectively, zero deductibles.

## Large-Deductible Plans Don't Work for the Chronically Sick

It is the chronically sick, obviously, who will suffer financially if they enroll in these newfangled defined-contribution policies. Sick people might save several hundred dollars annually in the form of lower premiums, but if they're incurring bills thousands of dollars in excess of their employer's contribution every year, they are worse off than they would have been under a more expensive policy with a more typical $500 deductible. I, and other critics of defined-contribution (DC) plans, have argued that these plans will, if they reach critical mass, drive the sick out of the market. They will do this by destroying non-DC plans.

This destruction will occur the way the "pod people" eliminated humanity in the movie, *Invasion of the Body Snatchers:* They will force non-DC companies to become like them, just as HMOs forced traditional insurers to mimic HMOs. The reason

DC plans will have the "pod people" effect on non-DC plans is that the non-DC plans will be stuck with sicker people, and this will force them to raise their premiums. The increase in premiums will cause another round of disproportionately healthy people to disenroll from the non-DC plans, which will force those plans to raise their premiums yet again, and around the vicious cycle will go. This cycle is known in the insurance industry as "a death spiral." A non-DC insurer caught in a death spiral will face two choices—die or become one of the pod people, that is, morph into a defined-contribution plan. The nation's largest HMOs are already offering DC plans, a sign that the HMOs are perfectly happy to adopt large-deductible policies if that's what it takes to survive.

> **❝** Fraud is reduced in single-payer systems because it is easier for one computer to detect fraud than it is for thousands of computers (belonging to thousands of private payers) to do so. **❞**

Large-deductible advocates are, by and large, hostile to managed care; they claim that the spread of DC plans will "empower consumers" and get managed care off our backs. But I have seen no indication that the insurance companies selling DC plans have sworn off managed care tactics. We are, in short, drifting toward the worst of all possible worlds—a world in which managed care policies with large deductibles dominate the market.

## Single-Payer System

A single-payer system refers to two reforms: replacing numerous insurers with one payer; and giving the one payer the authority to control prices charged by providers and drug companies. In the US today, multiple payers—1,000-plus insurance companies and dozens of government programs like Medicare, Medicaid and the VA—pay providers.

Nothing opens minds faster to the possibility that a single-payer with provider expenditure controls can reduce cost than a glance at per capita spending in industrialized nations. In 1998, the US, the only industrialized nation without a national health insurance system, paid $4,270 per person on health care. Switzerland, the nation with the world's second-most expensive system, paid only $2,740. The average expenditure for the industrialized world was about $2,000 per capita, less than half the US figure.

The insurance industry and its allies in politics and academia would have you believe that the rest of the industrialized world is paying a hideous price for their low expenditures. It is difficult to compare something as complex as national health care systems, but it is fair to say that the better funded national systems, such as those of Switzerland, Germany, France and Canada, are at least as good as America's system.

The data indicate, for example, that rationing is a much worse problem in the US than it is in Canada or Germany, that Canada has higher surgical survival rates than the US, and that Americans and Canadians get equally good cancer care. The one criticism of the Canadian system I have is that sporadic waiting lines for a few procedures have developed in some provinces. Although there is no scientific evidence that the small number of Canadians affected by delay in treatment that exceeds the US delay suffer damage to their health, there is little question that some of these patients suffer discomfort they shouldn't have to endure. To take a specific example, there is no evidence that the difference between the twelve-week delay for knee-replacement surgery in Canada and the five-week delay in the US causes harm to patients in either country. Nevertheless, Canadians with no cartilage in their knees spend an extra seven weeks living with their painful knees.

## Excessive Administrative Costs

If superior quality does not account for the extraordinary cost of the US system, what does? Answer: supply-side waste. Excessive administrative costs, excess capacity (which means too many hospital beds and too much equipment purchased to meet demand), excessively high prices, and fraud are the major categories of waste. Single-payer systems reduce excessive administrative costs by not wasting money on managing care, marketing, underwriting, lobbying, and profit. Excess capacity is addressed with budgets for hospitals; every year, hospitals negotiate a budget with the single-payer, and the single-payer sends a check to the hospital every month for one-twelfth of the negotiated budget. Every hospital may petition to buy its own burn unit, heart surgery unit, MRI, and helicopter, but not every hospital will get one. The single-payer (which, under the legislation COACT [Citizens Organized Acting Together] supported in Minnesota, would be a board of consumers) allows hospitals to purchase these things only if there is a need for them. Excessive physician fees and drug prices are eliminated with price controls. Fraud is reduced in single-payer systems because it is easier for one computer to detect fraud than it is for thousands of computers (belonging to thousands of private payers) to do so.

## Overuse and Underuse of Services

Note that I did not list "unnecessary services" as a form of waste. Advocates of HMOs and large deductibles stake their entire proposal on the premise that unnecessary services constitute the only or the primary source of waste in the system. It is true that unnecessary services are provided in this country (overuse of antibiotics is an example). However, underuse of the health care system is at least as prevalent as overuse. For example, half of all insured people with high blood pressure are not being treated for it. The solution to overuse is education of doctors and patients, not the large-deductible or HMO meat ax. Because the net of overuse and underuse is probably zero, and because a one-eyed focus on overuse has been used to justify HMOs and large deductibles, I don't list unnecessary services as a form of waste.

## A Single-Payer System Will Probably Be Implemented

Given the enormous power of the interests which oppose price controls and a single-payer system, it might seem like wishful thinking to predict that America will adopt price controls and a single-payer system. However, I think the odds are very high that we will impose price controls on all or a substantial portion of the health care industry within ten to 15 years, and I think the odds are good that we will implement a single-payer system, at either the national or state level, within the next ten to 30 years. I am optimistic on both price controls and single-payer for two reasons. First, polls and focus group sessions indicate that average citizens support single-payer by large margins when they are exposed to a fair debate about single-payer and other proposals. Second, the crisis is going to get worse, not better. That's because the health care industry, incapable of reforming itself, will continue to drive inflation up and quality down, and the aging of the Baby Boom generation will drive demand for health services to unprecedented levels over the next 30 years.

# 4

# Market-Based Plans Would Be Superior to a National Health Insurance Policy

## Merrill Matthews Jr.

*Merrill Matthews Jr. is a public policy analyst specializing in health care, Social Security, welfare, and Internet issues and is author of numerous studies in health policy. He is also director of the Council for Affordable Health Insurance, a Washington, D.C.–based research and advocacy organization promoting free-market insurance reform. In addition, he serves as medical ethicist for the University of Texas Southwestern Medical Center's Institutional Review Board for Human Experimentation. Matthews is a columnist for* Investor's Business Daily *and has published numerous articles in the* Wall Street Journal, USA Today, *and the* Washington Times.

The American health care system needs to function more like a business. Like other U.S. businesses, a for-profit medical business could provide high quality goods and services at affordable prices, something that critics of the business model argue can only be provided by nationalizing the health care system. Studies of the nationalized Canadian health care system show that quality has suffered significantly. For example, in Canada, patients wait in long lines to receive treatment, have limited access to new technology, and sometimes cannot get help at all. The United States would be making a mistake to adopt a nationalized health care system.

Merrill Matthews Jr. "Medicine as a Business," *The Mount Sinai Journal of Medicine*, vol. 71, September 2004, pp. 225–30. Copyright © 2004 by *The Mount Sinai Journal of Medicine*. Reproduced by permission.

Were this country beginning from scratch today, so that we had to consider separately each segment of the economic system and how it should work, many politicians and food policy experts surely would assert: Food is unique. And because it's unique, it could never be part of a free market system where consumers are free to make their own choices and vendors try to maximize profits.

Just consider, critics would assert, some of the problems that would arise if people could profit from the sale of food. We know that food is a necessity; everyone has to have it. Thus, consumers would be at the mercy of food producers, who could charge whatever they wanted to charge. Moreover, because there would be a financial incentive to keep costs as low as possible, food producers would constantly look for ways to cut quality. The result of these two forces would surely mean that consumers would pay very high prices for very low quality. And, of course, since most people aren't trained in nutrition, there would need to be an army of trained nutritionists to help them make good decisions.

> *The problems facing the health care system result not from its being too businesslike, but because the practice of medicine doesn't act enough like a business.*

Social thinkers helping to organize this new food system would point out that since humans must have food, it should be a basic human right. As a result, people without enough money to pay for their food should nevertheless be allowed to walk into a grocery store and take anything available without paying for it. These planners also might be concerned that under a free market system, higher-income individuals would be able to buy not only more but higher-quality food than those with low incomes, thus creating a two-tiered system. Such a situation, they might argue, is unfair and unjust. Do we really want a country in which some people have steak, while most settle for ground beef?

Their solution: raise taxes and use the increased government revenue to create a national food system that would ensure that everyone has equal access to food. Fortunately, we are not creating a food system from scratch. The one that has served us well for centuries operates almost completely under the free market system, and the result has been that the quality of food is high, the prices are low, and there is more than enough to go around. So why is it that people say that "medicine is unique" and want to do to the health care system what our food policy analysts might have done to the food system?

## The Business of Medicine

For the past several years there has been a growing debate among philosophers, ethicists, health care professionals and public policy analysts over whether medicine should function like a business, guided, as businesses are, by such worldly concerns as profits and customer satisfaction. Surely, they say, a profession as old, as self-sacrificing and as dedicated to the end of suffering and the betterment of humanity as medicine should be guided by some nobler, more altruistic goal.

Of course, the truth is that business permeates medicine— and big business at that. Health insurance and managed care companies, and the pharmaceutical and medical device industries are irrevocably intertwined with the health care system. Even doctors' practices are businesses; they pay rent, buy equipment, occasionally borrow money, meet payrolls and (usually) close out fiscal years with more income than outgo. Business is as important to medicine as new pharmaceuticals are to an effective physician: You just can't have one without the other. And most of those businesses are not confused about their priorities. They are there to help people, but they know that unless they make a profit, they won't be able to help people for long.

> *A single-payer system inherently tends to foster outdated medical techniques and resist new or innovative ones.*

Some doctors, as well as some philosophers, health policy analysts and visionaries, see medicine as a social endeavor. Physicians were meant to heal, not degrade themselves over paying rent, balancing books, fighting off lawsuits, justifying their decisions to managed care companies, or trying to keep

Congress from destroying the health care system.

Some physicians think medicine already looks too much like self-serving capitalism. Business is about taking care of yourself; medicine is about taking care of others. Business is guided by pragmatic decisions, medicine by ideals, and some physicians seek to take the business out of medicine so that the ideals can prevail. The idealists hope to do good without regard to doing well; the businesses in medicine strive to do well in order to continue doing good.

I will argue that, in contrast to such idealistic views, the problems facing the health care system result not from its being too businesslike, but because the practice of medicine doesn't act enough like a business. Business is guided by the very pragmatic goal of providing high quality goods and services to people, at affordable prices. Isn't that also the goal of medicine? Even those who think the government should run the health care system believe that. And they usually argue that nationalizing the health care system, thereby minimizing or completely eliminating the business element, will keep health care costs affordable while freeing doctors to provide quality health care. But is that what actually happens when a health care system is nationalized?

## Problems with Canada's Health Care System

Countries with national health care systems spend less on health care than does the U.S. For example, in 2001 the U.S. spent 13.9% of its gross domestic product (GDP), on health care, while Canada—a frequently cited "model" for U.S. reform—spent only about 9.7% of its GDP. But spending less on health care is not the only—and probably should not be the primary—goal. The challenge is to maintain a high-quality and responsive health care system while spending less money.

Has a country like Canada achieved that goal? The *New York Times* has revealed numerous problems all across Canada. According to one story:

- "[I]n Winnipeg, 'hallway medicine' has become so routine that hallway stretcher locations have permanent numbers. Patients recuperate more slowly in the drafty, noisy hallways, doctors report."
- At Vancouver General Hospital on the West Coast, "Maureen Whyte, a hospital vice president, estimates that 20 percent of heart attack patients who should have treat-

ment within 15 minutes now wait an hour or more."

- Finally, "Last summer [1999], as waiting lists for chemo-therapy treatments for breast and prostate cancer stretched to four months, Montreal doctors started to send patients 45 minutes down the highway to Champlain Valley Physicians' Hospital in Plattsburgh, New York."

As the *New York Times* points out, "Canada has moved informally to a two-tier, public-private system. Although private practice is limited to dentists and veterinarians, 90 percent of Canadians live within 100 miles of the United States, and many people are crossing the border for private care."

## A Flu Epidemic

A recent flu epidemic in Toronto expanded the waiting times to see a family physician to 5–6 weeks. Appointments were scheduled so far into the future that most patients would have recovered from their illness and would no longer have needed to see a doctor.

Unfortunately, many patients who needed to see a doctor immediately didn't even have an emergency room option. In December of 1999 and January of 2000, Toronto emergency rooms were so full that they were turning away patients—regardless of how sick they were. According to a story in the *Toronto Star*, 24 of 25 emergency rooms were closed on Monday, December 27, 1999. By the next day, "21 of 25 emergency wards were refusing to accept any new patients, no matter how ill or critically injured they might have been, or were accepting only the most serious cases." According to the authors, "Toronto Ambulance's paramedics were working the phones like veteran travel agents, trying to find emergency room spots for their patients on a day when the demand was close to its peak." Only three weeks later, an 18-year-old boy, Joshua Fleuelling, died of asthma because the emergency rooms were on "critical care bypass" and couldn't accept him.

## Waiting Lines

But it gets worse. In March of 2000, Canadian Health Minister Allan Rock told the House of Commons, "There are people who are waiting too long, waiting hours in the emergency ward, waiting months for referral to a specialist, waiting a year for a long-term bed, waiting what seems to be an eternity for someone to answer the call button in an understaffed hospital." Rock is referring to the Canadian health care system—one in which, according to supporters, accessibility, efficiency and affordability are all supposed to converge.

Canadians often wait weeks and even months to see a specialist. According to the Vancouver, British Columbia–based Fraser Institute's annual survey of waiting times in Canada:

- The average total waiting time between referral from a general practitioner and treatment by a specialist rose from 13.3 weeks in 1998 to 14 weeks in 1999.
- Waiting times between specialist consultation and treatment (which does not include the time between seeing a general practitioner and getting to see a specialist) increased from 7.3 weeks in 1998 to 8.4 weeks in 1999.
- Waiting times for diagnostic tests also underwent some increases. For example, the median wait for a CT scan across Canada was five weeks in 1999, a 6.4% increase over 1998.

## Canada's Budget Debate

In 2000, Canada's health care system reached a crisis over funding. In this case, however, the crisis wasn't instigated by budget deficits, but by a budget surplus. Some Members of Parliament wanted to pass an income tax cut of at least 20%, which others opposed, claiming that the proposed budget only offered two cents in health care funding for every dollar in tax cuts.

Ralph Klein, premier of Alberta, who wants to bring a little of the "business mindset" back into Canadian medicine by letting for-profit clinics perform some of the procedures currently provided by Canadian hospitals, has offered one solution to the problem of waiting lines. The government health care program, known as Medicare, would reimburse the clinics for the care.

## Limited Access to Technology

In a system where health care budgets are tight, bureaucrats and politicians tend to see new technology as too costly to justify the benefit they would provide. As a result, funds, if any, are provided only for the purchase of a limited amount of the newest technology. The decisions on what to buy and when to buy it are often arbitrary and guided more by good politics than good medicine.

Even more important, these arbitrary limits usually enshrine the medical knowledge and techniques current at a particular point in time. A central control system cannot afford new medical discoveries and treatments, because they aren't in the budget and no funding or other resources is allocated for them. Thus, a single-payer system inherently tends to foster outdated medical techniques and resist new or innovative ones.

> // *The current medical system distorts all of the normal incentives. Doctors do not believe that they are serving patients, but rather the insurers, the employers, the government or the managed care companies.* //

Although single-payer proponents cite Canada as a system that rivals the U.S. in the availability of new technology, the country lags behind many of the Organization for Economic Cooperation and Development (OECD) countries. While Canada ranks fifth in terms of total health care spending (as a percent of GDP), a recent study by the Fraser Institute, comparing OECD data, found that the country:

- Ranks 21 out of 28 in CT scanner availability;
- Is 19th out of 22 in lithotriptor availability;
- Is 19th out of 27 for the availability of MRIs.

Stories abound of Canadians going to extreme measures in order to gain access to medical technology. For example, several years ago an enterprising hospital in Guelph, Ontario, decided to allow animals needing computed tomography (CT) scans to enter the hospital in the middle of the night—charging pet owners $300 apiece. There is nothing necessarily wrong with that action, except that thousands of people in Ontario were waiting up to three months for an appointment on the same machine.

"I'd go any time," said Greg Moulton, who was in the middle of a two-month wait to learn why he was having "excruciating" headaches. Because people are not allowed to pay out of pocket for medical procedures covered under the government-run plan, they have to wait. However, if you're a dog, you can get medical technology immediately.

When dogs get better treatment than people, then people

will "become dogs." In December 1999, *The Washington Post* reported that waiting lines for magnetic resonance imaging (MRIs) in Ontario had grown so long that one Ontario resident "booked himself into a private veterinary clinic that happened to have one of the machines, listing himself as 'Fido.'"

## Rationing

At a 1999 conference in England organized by the Institute for Public Policy Research, Alan Milburn, health secretary of England, said of the country's National Health Service (NHS), "The NHS—just like every other health system in the world, public or private—has never, or will never, provide all the care it might theoretically be possible to provide. . . . So within our expanding health system there will always be choices to be made about the care to be provided."

Thus the question is, "Who decides about who gets what?" In a single-payer system, the government makes the larger decisions about funding levels, leaving the doctors, hospitals and other health care providers to make the tougher individual decisions about whose care to limit. The targets of rationing are usually the marginal cases, and that often means the very young, the very old and the very sick. The patient is often simply told, "There's nothing more we can do for you," a statement that is true within the confines of the budget. The range of medical options is simply not discussed in these circumstances.

The *Canadian Medical Association Journal* (CMAJ) reported in May 1999 that during a 12-month period, 121 patients waiting for coronary bypass surgery were removed from the waiting list because their conditions had deteriorated to the point where they were unlikely to survive surgery. "In Quebec," according to Steven Pearlstein of *The Washington Post*, "they've sent more than 250 cancer patients over the border to the United States this year (1999) to get treatment and still there are 350 who have waited more than four weeks for radiation or chemotherapy (waiting more than 4 weeks is considered medically risky)." Such stories are not rarities, but commonplace, even in the best of single-payer systems, and Canada is one of the best. The fact is that health care rationing is pervasive when the government controls health care. And as health care costs rise and government budgets tighten, rationing expands.

Canada has been very explicit about its attempt to avoid using the business model in health care. And this has led to waiting lines, increased pain and suffering, needless deaths, lack of access to technology and rationing. Is this really the model the U.S. should follow for providing quality health care?

## The Need to Get Incentives Right

The primary problem with the doctor-patient relationship as it exists today is that the incentives are complicated. In a market system, providers of goods and services know who they are try- ing to please—the customer—and why. It is in the interest of those who provide goods or services to make sure that their clients and customers are satisfied. A restaurant owner has an interest in making sure that those who come to his establish- ment enjoy their dinning experience. An attorney has an in- terest in ensuring that her clients are satisfied with her services.

This is not simply about economic interests. Most vendors want to have a good reputation for producing and selling qual- ity products. They want people to respect them for what they do and how they do it, not just for how much they make. For- tunately, those who develop a reputation for quality products or services usually get rewarded financially as well. When in- centives are operating properly, everyone walks away from a transaction happy—the vendor because he sold a product or service and made some money, and the customer because she has a product she wanted for a price she was willing to pay.

> *It is only by adopting the business model that medicine can embrace its values in providing a high level of quality for an affordable price.*

But who is the doctor trying to please? The patient or the managed care company or the employer? Most professionals have a fiduciary responsibility to their clients to work for their best interests. But to whom does the doctor owe a fiduciary re- sponsibility? Since the patient gets the care but the insurer pays the bill, it isn't clear exactly who the client/customer is.

The current medical system distorts all of the normal in- centives. Doctors do not believe that they are serving patients, but rather the insurers, the employers, the government or the managed care companies that are paying the patients' bills.

These managed care companies strive to disenroll those physicians who provide too much care. Patients aren't satisfied, because they feel that somebody is keeping them from getting the care they were promised and their employer paid for. And employers, insurers, state and federal governments, and managed care companies aren't happy, because they believe that doctors and patients are driving up health care spending and finding ways to sidestep or minimize the controls meant to keep health care costs low.

Consider just one of the perverse incentives common in the system. Under most circumstances, workers get paid more for doing more. But under a managed care capitation system, doctors get paid more for doing less. There is no way that this kind of incentive system will encourage satisfaction and confidence from either the patient or the physician.

## Making Medicine Work More Like a Business

The problems facing the health care system are not going to be resolved unless it begins to operate more like a business. That means getting the incentives right once again. The reason businesses seek to offer a quality product at an affordable price is that customers want value for their money. That is, they weigh cost, quality, service, convenience and other factors before making a decision on what to purchase.

To a large extent, customers in the health care system—otherwise known as patients—don't seek value for their dollars, because in the vast majority of cases they are spending someone else's money (i.e., the insurer's, the managed care company's, the employer's or the government's).

This insulation from the cost of health care has created a number of problems. When people are insulated from the cost of their economic decisions, they will spend more than they otherwise would. And the medical establishment has exacerbated the problem by pushing for everyone to be covered for everything. That is a prescription for financial disaster.

In addition, the tax system provides a generous tax break to those who get their health insurance through their employer, but not to those who buy it themselves. Because most employees think that employer money spent on health insurance comes from the employer—although most economists believe it is actually paid for by the employee because it is part of the total compensation package—they want their employer to buy as comprehensive a policy as possible. That practice has also contributed to the problem of people being overinsured.

## Using Major Medical Insurance

If people were to reduce some of that cost insulation—say, by choosing a high-deductible health insurance policy that covers them for a major accident or illness—they would begin to act more like consumers act in every other segment of the economy. If they were allowed to put the resulting savings in a tax-free account to pay for health care, they would be getting the same tax advantage they currently receive when the employer pays the health insurance bill. In fact, that is what flexible spending accounts (FSAs) and medical savings accounts (MSAs) are meant to do, but both plans are currently burdened by restrictions that have reduced their appeal.

Although it may seem radical, there is nothing new about this idea. Fifty years ago, health insurance was reserved almost exclusively for catastrophic medical events. It was even called "major medical." When patients visited a doctor, or the doctor came to their house, they paid those costs out of pocket. Of course, some patients didn't have the money and doctors had to work something out with them, perhaps by accepting a reduced fee or even nothing at all. The medical community's drive to make sure everyone has comprehensive health insurance has not resolved that problem. Doctors still have to reduce their prices, only now it's the managed care companies that are demanding the discounts.

Just imagine how much different the office visit would be if patients had to pay the full cost of, say, Celebrex or Vioxx out of their own funds or an MSA. Most would be much more interested than they are today in getting the doctor's opinion about whether the name brand or a less-expensive, over-the-counter pain reliever would do. That is where value would come in. Once patients are concerned about value, and health care providers are concerned about ensuring that patients receive that value, the proper incentives will be in place—and the health care system will begin to look a lot more like a successful business.

## Who Will Make Health Care Decisions?

There is no escaping it: someone will determine who gets what in health care. The question is whether that someone will be the patient in consultation with a doctor or some company overseeing health care costs.

For years many people both inside and outside the medical community have argued that "medicine is unique." And because it is unique, neither doctors nor patients should have to weigh the costs of health care with the benefits. As a result, managed care companies, employers, insurers and the government have stepped in and weighed those costs and made those decisions.

The medical profession will probably never operate completely like a business. Health insurance—even with a high deductible—will continue to insulate people from the full cost of care. And doctors will continue to provide care even to those who cannot afford it. But medicine can learn from business, and even become more like it. That means adjusting the incentives so that they create a positive, rather than a negative, impact.

In becoming more business oriented, medicine doesn't have to give up its own unique values. Indeed, it is only by adopting the business model that medicine can embrace its values in providing a high level of quality for an affordable price—just as the food system and most other businesses do.

# 5

# National Health Insurance Could Save Billions of Dollars

## David U. Himmelstein and Steffie Woolhandler

*David U. Himmelstein is an associate professor of medicine at Harvard and cofounder (with Steffie Woolhandler) of Physicians for a National Health Program (PNHP), an organization advocating for a single-payer national health insurance policy. Steffie Woolhandler is an associate professor of medicine at Harvard and codirector of the Harvard Medical School General Internal Medicine Fellowship program.*

A comprehensive study published in January 2004 estimated that national health insurance could save the United States at least $286 billion annually. High administrative spending in American health care is due to the excessive paperwork doctors and hospitals must deal with when working with hundreds of different insurance plans. By contrast, in Canada, where every patient has the same insurance, doctors fill out the same simple billing form for each patient, which is sent to one agency, saving Canadians massive amounts of money. Bureaucracy accounts for at least 31 percent of the total U.S. health spending whereas in Canada it is almost half that amount. The financial savings possible with a national health insurance plan such as Canada's could cover health care for all of America's uninsured, provide full prescription drug coverage for everyone in the country, and improve coverage and quality of care for those who already have insurance.

A study by researchers at Harvard Medical School and Public Citizen [a nonprofit consumer advocacy organization] finds that health care bureaucracy [in 2003] cost the United States $399.4 billion. The study estimates that national health insurance (NHI) could save at least $286 billion annually on paperwork, enough to cover all of the uninsured and to provide full prescription drug coverage for everyone in the United States.

The study was based on the most comprehensive analysis to date of health administration spending, including data on the administrative costs of health insurers, employers' health benefit programs, hospitals, nursing homes, home care agencies, physicians and other practitioners in the United States and Canada. The authors found that bureaucracy accounts for at least 31 percent of total U.S. health spending compared to 16.7 percent in Canada. They also found that administration has grown far faster in the United States than in Canada.

## What Savings Could Do

The potential administrative savings of $286 billion annually under national health insurance could:

1. Offset the cost of covering the uninsured (estimated at $80 billion)
2. Cover all out-of-pocket prescription drugs costs for seniors as well as those under 65 (estimated at $53 billion in 2003)
3. Fund retraining and job placement programs for insurance workers and others who would lose their jobs under NHI (estimated at $20 billion)
4. Make substantial improvements in coverage and quality of care for U.S. consumers who already have insurance

Looked at another way, the potential administrative savings are equivalent to $6,940 for each of the 41.2 million people uninsured in 2001 (the most recent figure available for the uninsured at the time study was carried out), more than enough to pay for health coverage. The study found wide variation among states in the potential administrative savings available per uninsured resident. Texas, with 4.96 million uninsured (nearly one in four Texans), could save a total of $19.5 billion a year on administration under NHI, which would make available $3,925 per uninsured resident per year. Massachusetts, which has very high per capita health administrative spending and a relatively low rate of uninsurance, could save a total of $8.6 billion a year, making available $16,453 per uninsured person. California, with 6.7 million uninsured, could save a total of $33.7 billion a year, which would make available $5,016 per uninsured person.

> *The study estimates that national health insurance (NHI) could save at least $286 billion annually on paperwork.*

[In early January 2004], the government reported that health spending accounts for a record 15 percent of the nation's economy and that health care spending shot up by 9.3 percent in 2002. Insurance overhead (one component of administrative costs) rose by a whopping 16.8 percent in 2002, after a 12.5 percent increase in 2001, making it the fastest growing component of health expenditure over the past three years. Hence the figures in the Harvard/Public Citizen Report (which was completed before release of these latest government figures) may understate true administrative costs.

## Factors Contributing to High Costs

The authors of the . . . study attributed the high U.S. administrative costs to three factors. First, private insurers have high overhead in both nations but play a much bigger role in the United States. Second, the United States fragmented payment system drives up administrative costs for doctors and hospitals, who must deal with hundreds of different insurance plans (for example, at least 755 in Seattle alone), each with different coverage and payment rules, referral networks, etc. In Canada, doctors bill a single insurance plan, using a single simple form, and hospitals receive a lump sum budget, much as a fire department is paid in the United States. Finally, the increasing business orientation of U.S. hospitals and insurers has expanded bureaucracy.

## Medicare Bill Will Increase Waste

The Medicare drug bill that Congress passed [in December 2003] will only increase bureaucratic spending because it will funnel large amounts of public money through private insurance plans with high overhead.

The recent Medicare bill means a huge increase in administrative waste and a big payoff for the AARP [American Association of Retired Persons]," said study author Dr. David Himmelstein, an associate professor of medicine at Harvard and former staff physician at Public Citizens Health Research Group. "At present, Medicare's overhead is less than 4 percent. But all of the new Medicare money, $400 billion, will flow through private insurance plans whose overhead averages 12 percent. So insurance companies will gain $36 billion from this bill. And the AARP stands to make billions from the 4 percent cut it receives from the policies sold to its members."

Dr. Steffie Woolhandler, a study author, associate professor of medicine at Harvard and a founder of Physicians for a National Health Program, said that hundreds of billions are squandered each year on health care bureaucracy, more than enough to cover all of the uninsured, pay for full drug coverage for seniors and upgrade coverage for the tens of millions who are underinsured. U.S. consumers spend almost twice as much per capita on health care as Canadians who have universal coverage and live two years longer. The administrative savings of national health insurance make universal coverage affordable.

> *Canadian hospitals do not bill individual patients for their care and so have no need to keep track of who receives each Band-Aid or an aspirin.*

Dr. Sidney Wolfe, director of Public Citizens Health Research Group added: "This study documents the state-by-state potential administrative savings achievable with national health insurance. These enormous sums could be used to provide health care for the more than 43 million uninsured people in the United States and drug coverage for seniors. These data should awaken governors and legislators to a fiscally sound and humane way to deal with ballooning budget deficits. Instead of cutting Medicaid and other vital services, officials could expand services by freeing up the $286 billion a year wasted on administrative expenses. In the current economic climate, with unemployment rising, we can ill afford massive waste in health care. Radical surgery to cure our failing health insurance system is sorely needed."

## The Simpler Canadian System

Dr. Himmelstein described the real-world meaning of the difference in administration between the United States and Canada by comparing hospitals in the two nations. Several years ago, he visited Toronto General Hospital, a 900-bed tertiary care center that offered an extensive array of high-tech procedures, and searched for the billing office. It was hard to find, though; it consisted of a handful of people in the basement whose main job was to send bills to U.S. patients who had come across the border. Canadian hospitals do not bill individual patients for their care and so have no need to keep track of who receives each Band-Aid or an aspirin.

"A Canadian hospital negotiates its annual budget with the provincial health plan and receives a single check each month to cover virtually all of its expenses," Himmelstein said. "It need not fight with hundreds of insurance plans about whether each day in the hospital was necessary, and each pill justified. The result is massive savings on hospital billing and bureaucracy."

Doctors in Canada face a similarly simple billing system. Every patient has the same insurance. There is one simple billing form with a few boxes on it. Doctors check the box indicating what kind of visit they provided to the patient (i.e., how long and whether any special procedures were performed) and send all bills to one agency.

## American Doctors Face Billing Nightmares

Himmelstein returned to Boston and visited Massachusetts General Hospital, which was similar to Toronto General in size and in the range of services provided. Himmelstein was told that Massachusetts General's billing department employed 352 full-time personnel, not because the hospital was inefficient, but because this department needed to document in detail every item used for each patient and fight with hundreds of insurance plans about payment.

U.S. doctors face a similar billing nightmare, Himmelstein said. "They deal with hundreds of plans, each with different rules and regulations, each allowing physicians to prescribe a different group of medications, each dictating that doctors refer patients to different specialists."

The U.S. system is a paperwork nightmare for doctors and patients, and wastes hundreds of billions of dollars.

# 6

# Personal Health Plans Are the Best Solution to America's Health Care Crisis

## Devon M. Herrick

*Devon M. Herrick is a policy expert and a senior fellow at the National Center for Policy Analysis (NCPA), a nonprofit, nonpartisan research organization. Herrick concentrates on health care issues such as Internet-based medicine, health insurance, the uninsured, and pharmaceutical drug issues. He has conducted several major research projects for the NCPA and has published several research studies and papers on health policy. In addition, he is a speaker on health policy issues.*

Personal health accounts are tax-free savings accounts that individuals use to pay medical expenses. Personal health accounts allow patients to purchase the health services they prefer rather than those chosen for them by their employer or insurance company. Lower income workers and the uninsured are attracted to these plans because, much like a savings account, money can accumulate in personal health accounts and be used for future health problems. Because any money in the account that is not used can be saved and utilized to cover future costs, patients tend to be more discretionary when deciding whether to go to the doctor, resulting in better control of health care costs.

When Medicare was first created, over 30 years ago, nobody anticipated that prescription drugs would become such an important part of health care, and thus, Congress did not think to include prescription drugs in the benefits offered under the program. Congress is busy trying to negotiate a bill to fix the oversight in the government's coverage for senior citizens [the bill passed]. This effort to update the program, however, is itself somewhat antiquated. Today, the market for health insurance is moving away from "one size fits all" group plans toward plans that give individual consumers and families greater control over the resources spent on their behalf.

Such plans often referred to as "consumer-driven insurance" allow individuals to control their own tax-free savings accounts to be used in paying for medical expenses or buying insurance. Many economists and health-care experts predict these plans will soon replace managed care as the next big health insurance initiative. If so, they offer an opportunity for reforming not just the tax treatment of private insurance, but for reforming Medicare as well. Simply put, seniors who control their own health-care resources don't need to worry about whether Congress acts to add a prescription drug benefit.

Approximately 88% of Americans with private health insurance are insured through their jobs, but there is a crisis of rising health insurance premiums. In addition, there is an employee backlash against the rationing of care by third parties, such as managed care providers.

Consumer-driven plans may account for as much as half of the market for employer-sponsored health insurance within the next four years. This would be a truly amazing development, considering that less than 1% of U.S. workers (fewer than 1.5 million) are currently enrolled in these plans.

## Medical Savings Accounts

The renewed interest in Medical Savings Accounts has caused some insurance firms to roll out products to capitalize on expected growth in the individual market for health insurance. In addition, the market for individual health insurance is expected to grow as a result of Bush administration proposals to use tax credits to help individuals buy policies.

This will be especially true if more employers reduce or eliminate coverage for workers' family members. Currently, nearly 7% of the insured population in the United States (more than 16 million people) buy their own health insurance policies rather than obtaining coverage through work.

Why all the brouhaha over health insurance? For one thing, prices have (again) begun to rise at double-digit annual rates. Managed care held down costs for a while, but many experts believe further restraint is unlikely.

The problem in health care is that, in most cases, medical services are free (or cost little) at the point of service. So consumers and doctors have the incentive to use as many services as the health insurers will pay for. This is very inefficient, since patients would consume fewer medical services (and pay less for health care) if most incidental medical services were paid out-of-pocket rather than through an "all you can eat buffet" managed-care model.

> **The problem in health care is that, in most cases, medical services are free (or cost little) at the point of service.**

Managed care was supposed to counter this tendency by telling patients which medical services they needed and could have. That caused a backlash in much the same way a restaurant buffet would go bankrupt if the owner tried to tell patrons how much they were allowed to eat.

However, if patients control a portion of the money used to pay incidental medical services and get to keep a proportion of any money saved, then the incentive to overindulge would be cut back sharply. Economists know this. In a recent poll, for example, two-thirds of the members of the National Association of Business Economics (NABE) said that consumer-driven health insurance is either very important or extremely important in controlling costs, improving access and increasing health-care quality.

Many insurance industry experts agree. A survey of insurance industry experts by Gabel et al., in *Health Affairs Market Watch* predicts that consumer-driven health plans will account for 20% of the health insurance market by 2005, and as much as 50% by 2007. In addition, BNA [Bureau of National Affairs] reports that consumer-driven plans will account for at least 24% of the health insurance market by 2010.

Employers providing a consumer-driven health plan deposit a portion of the insurance premiums into an account controlled by employees. This allows employees to buy medical services at their discretion. These personal health accounts are usually coupled with a high-deductible, catastrophic policy that covers serious medical events above the amount in the personal health savings account. This contrasts sharply with managed care, where (once premiums have been paid) most medical services and drugs are free at the point of service.

Currently there are three types of personal health accounts that make up consumer-driven health insurance plans. These are: medical savings accounts (MSAs), flexible spending accounts (FSAs) and health reimbursement arrangements (HRAs). Each option provides patients with tools to be empowered medical consumers by controlling a greater portion of their health spending. Unfortunately, each option also has limitations. . . .

## Patient Power

Consumer-driven health insurance plans that feature personal health accounts, like MSAs and HRAs (and to some extent FSAs), allow patients to purchase the health services they prefer, not those chosen for them by an employer or an insurance company. They are also very popular with employees because of their flexibility. For instance, a patient purchasing health care from a personal health account does not need to seek prior approval before seeing a specialist. Nor do patients face obstacles if they wish to use alternative-care providers.

Healthy workers aren't the only ones to benefit from MSAs and HRAs. In fact, those with chronic illnesses benefit because their health-care needs are greater. Health insurance plans that allow patients greater flexibility to decide the types of health care that best address specific conditions are exactly what chronically ill patients need. . . .

## Advantages of Health Accounts

Health-care savings accounts have been shown to be powerful tools to control health-care costs. In South Africa, where half of privately insured workers are enrolled in MSAs, studies show that patients with MSAs cut discretionary spending by more than 50%. In addition, research on the South African experience by the National Center for Policy Analysis shows that patients with MSAs do not skimp on preventive care.

MSA patients also are not deprived of discounts available to large insurers. In almost all MSA plans, patients spending their own MSA money are entitled to the very same discounts that their insurer pays, as long as they stay in the network. And even when they go out of network, they often get big discounts from doctors who welcome patients paying cash.

> **// Health-care savings accounts have been shown to be powerful tools to control health-care costs. //**

An often-used criticism of personal health accounts is they would favor the wealthy, who might use them as a way to shelter funds tax-free far beyond what might be needed for medical needs. In reality, MSAs and HRAs are seldom used as tax shelters. And with many Americans getting older, it only makes sense to encourage saving for future medical needs.

Employer-paid health insurance premiums are already excluded from taxation. And, as policy wonks point out, this tax subsidy already benefits higher-income workers more than low-income workers. If we hope to level the playing field and give low-income workers a chance to obtain coverage that doesn't penalize them in the event they don't need care, they need access to personal health accounts. Otherwise, many low-income workers would forgo health insurance.

Moreover, these accounts need to be tax free. Currently, tax law encourages us to give all our health dollars to an insurer and endure an HMO form of health-care delivery. Exempting consumer-driven accounts from taxes places them on a level playing field with employer-sponsored health insurance plans. Furthermore, a RAND Corporation study found that families choosing MSAs had lower incomes and greater health-care needs than those who chose managed care. The liberal Urban Institute reached a similar conclusion.

## Help for the Uninsured

Finally, MSAs significantly reduce the number of uninsured. The IRS reports 73% of the 100,000 current MSA holders previously had no insurance. MSAs make health insurance more attractive to the uninsured because they get to keep the money they don't spend. Census figures show that 41% of the uninsured (i.e., almost 18 million people) are young people between the ages of 18 and 34. Data from the Bureau of Labor Statistics illustrate that these people tend to spend far more money on dining away from home and entertainment than on out-of-pocket health care.

It is likely that many of these people are healthy and don't consider health insurance to be a good buy. The reason they may prefer to spend their money on goods and services other than health insurance might be because they don't think they are likely to need medical care beyond what they can pay out of pocket and don't want to subsidize older (often wealthier) workers. More younger workers might consider health insurance a good buy if they could roll over a substantial portion of their premiums to accumulate and grow for future years when health needs might be greater.

Personal health accounts such as MSAs, HRAs and FSAs . . . will continue to grow and offer consumers the power to choose the health care that meets their needs. Research has shown that employees are more satisfied when they have greater choice of plans and consumer-driven health care offers them the ultimate choice.

An important by-product is that the quality of health care and service improves when patients are the ones who control the checkbook, rather than third-party insurers. Another important result is that costs will rise more slowly. Over 100 million consumers holding a tight rein on health-care spending will do more to control costs than a few third-party bureaucrats working for HMOs.

# 7

# America Should Model Its Health Care System After Those of Other Developed Nations

## Rudolph Mueller

*Rudolph Mueller is a physician, and an assistant professor of medicine at the State University of New York in Buffalo. He is also a fellow of the American College of Physicians.*

In every industrialized, democratic country except the United States health care is recognized as a human right and is provided to individuals regardless of economic class. Although many Americans believe that the United States has exceptional health care, the truth is that it is mediocre. It ranks twenty-fourth out of 191 countries in health or the provision of good health. People in other countries such as Great Britain, Canada, Spain, Germany, and France enjoy higher life expectancies, more years without disability, lower infant mortality rates, and greater patient satisfaction. In the United States, where a large health care underclass exists, the gap between the rich and the poor is widening, creating even greater disparity in health care service. Examining the health care systems of other countries can provide models for much needed reform.

Evaluating the healthcare systems and policies of other nations is important in determining the strong and weak points of our own system. . . . In every other industrialized democratic country of the world, healthcare is a validated human right. The intention of those governments is to provide for the well-being and dignity of individuals of every economic class. In the United States, however, there is a large healthcare underclass. . . . An OECD [Organization for Economic Cooperation and Development] survey showed that only 45% of Americans have guaranteed health insurance.

Most OECD countries guarantee health insurance for nearly 100% of their population, while realizing the importance of the caregivers (doctors, nurses, and hospitals) and pharmaceutical companies. It is in these countries' experiences that we should seek a structure for healthcare for the United States. All that is British in healthcare is not necessarily bad. All that is French is not necessarily good.

For the elite of America and the fully insured, the treatment available may be the best in the world. But the system fails so many others and leaves a massive underclass of patients. Continuing our present system is far too expensive and incredibly unjust.

[Founder of the German Empire] Otto von Bismarck inaugurated the first healthcare program in the world for German citizens in the newly unified nation in 1883 as part of an embryonic social contract. Starting in the 1940s and continuing through the 1970s, European countries provided and guaranteed a basic level of universal care to their citizens. For virtually all Europeans, healthcare delivery to the patient is based on medical need.

> *Continuing our present system is far too expensive and incredibly unjust.*

These countries, that provide universal healthcare coverage, have dramatically lower overall costs. Their people enjoy higher life expectancy, more years without disability, lower infant mortality rates, and greater general patient satisfaction compared to the United States. The U.S. continues to demonstrate the mediocre overall health of its people. I believe this is unsatisfactory for this great nation. According to a 1998 Commonwealth Fund Survey, 28% of Americans found it "extremely," "very," or "somewhat difficult" to get medical care when needed compared to 21% in Canada and 15% in Australia and Great Britain. Americans had six physician visits per year per capita compared to 6.5 in Germany and France, 6.6 in Australia and 6.8 in Canada. In 1997, Americans had the shortest hospital stays compared to all OECD countries at 7.3 hospital days compared to 9.8 in Great Britain, 8.4 in Canada, 10.0 in France and Australia, and 12.5 in Germany. Recently, I saw one of my patients after he had heart bypass surgery and he told me his hospital stay was only three and a half days. Thankfully, he did well; others have not.

> *All Americans have the right to decent healthcare and should be treated appropriately regardless of their ability to pay.*

According to a recent study, bypass patients have seen significantly shorter hospital stays averaging 5.4 in 1998 versus 9.2 days in 1990. Unfortunately, in 1998 patients were ten times more likely to be readmitted and 15 times more likely to be transferred to an extended care facility with an average length of stay being 10.6 days.

## Disparities Between Rich and Poor

In Canada, the cost of healthcare to families of different incomes is skewed so that the wealthier share more of the burden. In the United States that skew is reversed. The poor pay more for care as a percentage of income. Even in countries with universal care, the poor continue to have worse outcomes compared to the rich. This disparity between rich and poor is profound. Part of the disparity is the economic and societal pressures placed on the poor, sick patients.

In a society with a large income gap between the rich and the poor, citizens die at a higher rate compared to people living in more equitable societies. Some refer to and measure this gap as the "Robin Hood index" which relates to the size of income differences between the rich and the poor. . . . This income gap and its relationship to overall mortality of a population have also been demonstrated in other studies.

In the U.S., the wealthiest nation in the world in GDP [gross domestic product] per capita at purchasing power parity, there is a wide and continually growing gap between the rich and the poor. From 1960 to 1986 overall mortality rates fell, but more significantly for the rich and well educated, and less so for the poor and less-educated Americans. Then the economic boom in the 1990s supposedly benefited all Americans, but most of the significant gains went to those in the top 20%. Those in the middle groups may actually have become worse off financially during those prosperous times. Another report from a 1999 Public Policy Institute of California study showed that Californians' family income at the 10th percentile (inflation adjusted) dropped 14%, from $15,810 in 1969 to $13,600, while those in the 90th percentile increased 58%, from $86,140 in 1969 to $135,850. I believe these large gaps between the rich and the poor contribute to the poor health of individuals and our society. I believe all Americans have the right to decent healthcare and should be treated appropriately regardless of their ability to pay. . . .

All of the developed countries of the world provide care at significantly lower costs in terms of percentages of gross domestic product compared to the U.S. In 1997, per capita spending on total healthcare services was $4,090 in the U.S., while the median for the twenty-nine OECD countries was $1,747.

## How the United States Ranks

The 2000 World Health Organization Review of 191 nations ranked the United States as thirty-seventh overall in health system performance, but number one in healthcare costs at 13.7% of GDP or $4,187 per capita in spending. We were also judged to be first in responsiveness to the expectations of the population, including respect for the dignity of individuals, confidentiality of health records, prompt attention in emergencies and widest choice of providers. Despite this "responsiveness," we only ranked twenty-fourth in health or the provision of good health (as measured by life expectancy adjusted for the likelihood of a range of disabilities). The average American has 4.5 years less of good health compared to the citizens of top ranking Japan. We also rated low, at fifty-fourth, in financial fairness or the fairness of individuals' financial contribution toward their health as measured by the equal distribution of the health costs among households. . . .

Great Britain and Spain are examples of government operated national health services in which doctors and others are mostly salaried. In Britain there are also private hospitals and private insurance for those who wish it.

In a "single-payer" national health insurance system, as in Canada, Denmark, Sweden, and Australia, insurance is publicly administered, and most physicians are in private practice.

Highly regulated, universal multi-payer health insurance systems are in place in countries like Germany, France, The Netherlands, Italy and Japan, which have universal health insurance via sickness funds or similar mechanisms. These funds pay physicians and hospitals uniform rates that are negotiated annually. Also known as an "all-payer" system, participation in the funds is mandatory, which makes them essentially funded by the government and taxpayers. Physicians not on hospital or university staffs are in private practice. . . .

The United States . . . has no national healthcare policy. Every other industrialized nation has one based on the United Nations Declaration of 1948.[1] Without a national policy things get out of hand.

---

1. The 1948 United Nations Universal Declaration of Human Rights, Article 25, says that "Everyone has the right to a standard of living adequate for the health and well being of himself and his family, including food, clothing, housing, and medical care."

# 8

# Employer-Based Insurance Leaves Many Uninsured

## Leif Wellington Haase and Cari Reiner

*Leif Wellington Haase is a fellow of the Century Founda-
tion, an institution that works as a think tank providing information on national issues. Haase's areas of expertise are
health care, homeland security, and retirement security. He
is the staff director of the Century Foundation's task force on
Medicare reform. Haase has also written numerous articles
on health care in publications including the* Boston Globe
*and the* American Prospect Online, *and has given commentaries on National Public Radio. Cari Reiner works as an
intern for the* Century Foundation Research.

More than 60 percent of Americans receive health insurance through their employment, making the
United States the only industrialized nation where the
majority of citizens obtain health insurance through
their jobs. Those who cannot get insurance through
their employers, and who are not eligible for Medicare
or Medicaid, must either pay for their own health insurance or forgo coverage altogether. As of 2002, an estimated 43 million Americans, or 15 percent of the
population, were uninsured. The large number of
uninsured Americans creates problems for everyone.
For example, the uninsured are less likely to receive
preventive services such as vaccinations, increasing the
chance that infectious diseases will spread much more
quickly. Clearly, the present employer-based system
does not work for many Americans.

A lone among developed nations, the United States relies primarily on employers to provide health insurance for its citizens. More than 60 percent of Americans obtain medical coverage as a benefit from their own jobs or from family members' jobs. Citizens aged sixty-five and older are entitled to federal Medicare coverage, and some low-income Americans are eligible for Medicaid. But most others whose employers do not provide health insurance either must pay for their own costly coverage or gamble that they will not face major medical bills.

This employer-based system is the principal reason why such a large portion of the population lacks health insurance. As of 2002, 43.6 million Americans under the age of sixty-five—more than 15 percent of the population—had no medical coverage. Since the mid-1970s, the number of uninsured has increased at an average rate of almost 1 million per year.

Ten years ago [in 1994], the Clinton administration put forth a proposal for universal health care that tried to loosen the link between employment and health insurance. Congress rejected the proposal. Evidence suggests that the problem of increasing numbers of uninsured Americans will continue as long as the nation's health care system is reliant on employers voluntarily offering insurance.

## A Swiss Cheese System

Employer-based health insurance coverage in the United States developed through a combination of historical circumstances, policy decisions, and expedience. A relatively modern phenomenon, private coverage grew rapidly during World War II, when companies faced wage and price controls and competed for labor by offering generous benefits, including health insurance. After the war, tax law evolved so that employees would not have to claim those benefits as taxable income and corporations could deduct insurance costs from their taxable earnings. These laws, which labor unions strongly supported and remain committed to, were in effect subsidies that encouraged employers to offer health insurance coverage.

Nevertheless, large numbers of employed Americans do not benefit from employment-based coverage because of the following weaknesses in the system:

- *Employees in small businesses are much less likely to be offered coverage than those who work for large companies (businesses with more than two hundred employees).* The cost per employee of health insurance is generally lower for large companies because risk is spread among a broader pool of workers. More than a quarter of all working-age Americans in companies with fewer than twenty-five employees are uninsured. These workers account for almost half the total number of uninsured Americans who are employed.

- *Layoffs and job switching lead to irregular and episodic insurance coverage.* The Congressional Budget Office estimates that 21 million to 31 million Americans go without coverage for a full year or more, while 57 million to 59 million are without coverage at some point during a given year.

- *Part-time and temporary workers are more likely to be uninsured.* According to the Kaiser Commission on Medicaid and the Uninsured, 31 percent of Americans in households with only part-time workers are uninsured, compared to 18 percent in households with one full-time worker and just 8 percent in households with two full-time workers. This situation looks even more troubling in light of the growing trend for companies to hire temporary workers and consultants to whom they do not offer health and other job benefits.

- *Nearly one in three young adults between the ages of nineteen and twenty-four lack health insurance.* Younger Americans are most likely to be uninsured because they either are unemployed, have episodic employment, or forgo coverage since they expect to be in good health.

- *A substantial percentage of minorities do not have health benefits.* Hispanics (7.7 percent) and African Americans (10.8 percent) have higher unemployment rates than whites (5.2 percent) and are more likely to be employed in jobs without benefits. Their employment status is one reason minorities are more likely to lack health care coverage than whites.

## Increased Pressure on Employers

Because health insurance costs for employers continue to rise rapidly—their premiums rose 13.9 percent on average between 2002 and 2003, far outpacing inflation and growth in wages—some companies have dropped employee coverage entirely. The percentage of employers offering health insurance to current workers declined from 69 percent to 66 percent between 2000 and 2003.

Among companies that provide coverage, the percentage of total costs paid by the employer has remained steady. But, both employers and workers are spending more and more on health insurance every year, which puts increasing pressure on employers to reduce benefits and require higher contributions from workers.

> **" Because health insurance costs for employers continue to rise rapidly . . . some companies have dropped employee coverage entirely. "**

One case in point is Wal-Mart, the nation's largest private employer, which has dropped retiree coverage, instituted a six-month waiting period for benefits for new hourly employees, and declined to pay for flu shots, childhood vaccinations, and other preventive services. Wal-Mart, which cut health care costs to around 60 percent of the average for large companies, may well become a model for other large firms.

## Everybody's Problem

The absence of health insurance coverage harms individuals and has profound social and economic consequences. Individuals without health insurance typically are billed higher amounts than insured Americans for their health care services because health insurance companies have the ability to negotiate prices. Uninsured Americans also are more likely than the insured to use emergency rooms, one of the most expensive sites to receive treatment, for routine care.

Individuals without insurance are less likely to see a physician, to have a regular source of care, to use preventive medical services, or to receive treatment for chronic conditions. Lack of access to such care can have damaging effects on health. Treatable diseases and conditions, such as diabetes, can go undiagnosed in early stages and worsen by the time an uninsured patient seeks care. Moreover, the uninsured receive less appropriate care, based on treatment guidelines, than that obtained by insured Americans. A study commissioned by the Institute of Medicine concluded that 18,000 deaths among adults aged twenty-five to sixty-four are directly attributable each year to the lack of insurance coverage.

The problem of the uninsured affects all Americans, regardless of their insurance status. On average, uninsured individuals pay only 35 percent of their medical expenses in a given year. The remainder of this cost is borne by public and private payers and by federal, state, and local taxpayers. In 2001, approximately $40 billion of uncompensated care—that is, care not paid for out of pocket or by private or public insurance—was provided, three-quarters of it funded by federal and state governments.

A large uninsured population puts everyone's health at greater risk. Because the uninsured are less likely to receive preventive services such as vaccinations, an outbreak of an infectious disease such as measles or whooping cough can spread much more quickly. Moreover, hospitals have been forced to cut other programs to make up for the costs of treating uninsured patients.

> *A study commissioned by the Institute of Medicine concluded that 18,000 deaths among adults aged twenty-five to sixty-four are directly attributable each year to the lack of insurance coverage.*

Finally, American companies face a unique burden in their competition with foreign counterparts because they bear the brunt of paying for the health care costs of their workers. Executives at DaimlerChrysler told the *Washington Post* that their worker health care costs per vehicle produced were in the $1,200–$1,300 range for a midsize car, about twice the cost of the sheet metal in the automobile. Health costs per employee in the United States are about ten times those in Canada, where income and sales taxes fund a universal single-payer system.

## Possible Cures

Only three of the Organisation for Economic Co-operation and Development (OECD) nations—Mexico, Turkey, and the United States—lack universal or near-universal coverage. Some proposals for universal health insurance coverage would attempt to expand employer coverage. Others, such as a single-payer system, would phase it out. Some of the most commonly discussed models for reform include:

- *Expanding Public Programs and Offering a Tax Credit.* This reform would merge existing public programs (Medicare, Medicaid, and the State Children's Health Insurance Program), expand their scope, and offer a tax credit for moderate-income Americans toward the purchase of health insurance.
- *Employer and Individual Mandates.* Building on existing employment-based insurance, this proposal would mandate employers to cover all employees and require employees to take this coverage. Premium subsidies would be offered to certain employers to enable them to afford the coverage they offer their employees.
- *Individual Mandates with Tax Credits.* Under this model, the responsibility for obtaining health insurance would rest with individuals. Individuals and families would receive tax credits to help them purchase health insurance.
- *Single Payer.* In this scenario, the federal government would collect and disburse all payments for health care, set uniform benefit packages, and create policies and standards for participation by providers and provider systems. Private insurance would be effectively eliminated.

While any of these models conceivably might improve on the current health system, none of them are likely to solve entirely the problems of cost and access that bedevil employer-based coverage. To retain or expand employer coverage probably would require very large subsidies. In all likelihood, the plans based on tax credits will not offer credits large enough to purchase good and affordable coverage in most areas. A Canadian-style, single-payer plan probably would end employer coverage but would radically disrupt the current system of private insurance coverage. It also could stifle medical innovation if the government refused to pay for expensive new treatments.

## A Plan Like Congressional Members Have

One alternative would be to eliminate the current tax breaks for employer-based coverage, to consolidate government-run health insurance programs, to seek other sources of savings (such as gains, over time, from improved public health), and then to use this redirected money to subsidize individual and family-purchased coverage. This could eventually give every American access to excellent basic coverage. Those who wanted more elaborate care would pay higher insurance premiums. In some respects, this model of coverage would resemble the one that members of Congress currently enjoy.

# 9

# Insurance Companies Limit Necessary Medical Care

## George D. Lundberg

*George D. Lundberg is editor in chief and executive vice president of Medscape, a provider of medical information on the Internet. Lundberg was editor for the* Journal of the American Medical Association (JAMA) *for seventeen years and is on the faculties of Northwestern University in Chicago and the School of Public Health at Harvard. He has published many articles in scientific journals and the popular press and appears regularly on national television.*

At the core of health care problems today is the fact that medical services and procedures are dictated by insurance companies. If a patient's insurance covers a procedure, it is performed; if insurance does not cover the procedure, it tends not to be performed. This practice has had devastating repercussions for patients. Indeed, numerous patients have died because they did not get the tests and treatments they needed on time.

S ome years ago a patient named Cynthia Herdrich of Urbana, Illinois, was forced to wait eight days for an ultrasound examination. Her health plan made the decision after her doctor examined her for abdominal pain. During the wait her appendix burst, and she underwent more complicated, extensive, and potentially risky surgery for peritonitis. Subsequently she filed suit against the health plan.

Inga Petrovich had to wait one year for an MRI [magnetic resonance imaging] when her health plan denied her physician's initial request. The delayed test revealed cancer at the base of her tongue, a cancer that eventually resulted in her death. Donna Marie McIlwaine of Scottsville, New York, was denied a proper diagnostic workup by her plan when her doctor examined her for chest pain and shortness of breath. She died within a week from pneumonia and a blood clot in her left lung—clearly treatable conditions.

Of course, in each of these cases the patient could have offered to pay for the test herself, or the physician or institution could have done the procedure without insurance company approval. However, patients typically don't pay for services out of pocket, and physicians and institutions typically don't move without insurance approval.

## What Is Wrong with the Health Care System

And that is precisely what is wrong with the current health care system. Insurance coverage decisions should be made by the medical profession and by a fully informed public. The profession should be responsible for restraining the overuse of expensive medical services, and proven preventive measures should be available without question. The profession and the public should be involved in establishing reasonable health care budgets and living within them in a regionally organized system. Instead, all of these decisions are being made by employers, insurers, managed care companies, and government officials.

> *More than 30 million people who have insurance are seriously and significantly underinsured.*

How did this happen? It's a long story, very like the one about the development of health insurance. Like that story, it also is filled with good intentions and bad results. One of the worst results is that medical services and procedures tend to follow insurance coverage. That is, procedures covered by insurance generally are performed, while procedures not covered by insurance tend not to be performed, or at least not frequently.

That practice is at the core of the many problems that so many people are having with health care today. The massive number of insurance restraints on coverage now in place are rigorously enforced. Only a few years ago the doors to medical care seemed to be wide open. Now more and more of them seem to be closed, and almost every day we see another newspaper story about a disaster flowing from insurance denials of medical care. Even when UnitedHealth Group announced that it would no longer routinely require preauthorization for most physician orders, physician autonomy was not restored in any clear-cut fashion. We are beginning to understand, in an entirely new way, that health insurance does not always ensure access to needed services.

> **" The vast majority of those with insurance now are enrolled in some type of managed care plan. "**

Of the more than 280 million people in the United States, all but 44 million are covered by some form of health insurance. Of the insured, approximately 39 million are covered by Medicare, 35 million by Medicaid, and the remainder by some form of employment-based insurance. But more than 30 million people who have insurance are seriously and significantly underinsured. They do not have the kind of comprehensive, in-depth coverage that studies have shown results in more timely medical care and better outcomes. Stated another way, the statistics indicate that only a minority of our population is covered by adequate, employment-based insurance.

## The Benefits of Comprehensive Insurance

People with comprehensive insurance are more likely to get what they need when they need it, and they are more likely to recover safely and quickly from medical interventions. By contrast, the uninsured and underinsured may delay seeing the doctor because they have either no insurance or a high deductible. They also may arrive sicker than those with good coverage, and they may experience more difficult and troublesome recoveries from medical treatments. Furthermore, they may bankrupt themselves if their lifetime insurance limits are too low.

But comprehensive insurance, such as that offered by traditional fee-for-service insurers, is hard to find today. In 1988, 71 percent of workers and families were covered by fee-for-service plans. That figure dropped to 49 percent in 1993, had plummeted to 30 percent by 1995, and continues to fall. The vast majority of those with insurance now are enrolled in some type of managed care plan.

Furthermore, more than 50 million people with managed care insurance are in plans that are not regulated by state insurance departments because they are preempted by federal law. Enacted in 1974, the Employee Retirement and Income Security Act (ERISA) was designed to protect pension plans, but employers who decided to self-insure also gained freedom from state insurance regulators under the act. Large multisite employers complained that their health benefits programs were uneven and difficult to manage because of variations in state regulations.

ERISA was supposed to ensure consistency, but what it really ensured was a free hand for employers and a significant loss of control over health decisions by employees. The latter soon discovered that they lived in a netherworld in which the rules were made, and changed at will, by their employers. This is a different kind of underinsurance because the limits of coverage are not spelled out in the insurance policy. Instead, they are determined by faceless administrators making decisions from remote locations about individual patients' medical needs.

Predictably horror stories such as those at the beginning of this [viewpoint] emerged from this kind of insurance coverage and began working their way through the courts. Patients and physicians now seem caught in a new system of health insurance coverage that neither group likes. Both are keenly aware that insurance itself does not guarantee good patient care. What the patient wants and what the doctor thinks often no longer seem to matter, and resolution of this problem promises to be the focus of an intense political debate as the new Congress and new administration take office in [2001].

What they will discover as they dig into the issues of coverage is the deeper issue at the core of medicine: Is it a business, a profession, or some sort of ongoing mixture of both? Which set of values will guide decisionmaking about the coverage of medical services?

# 10

# Health Care Fraud Is a Serious Problem

## Angela Maas

*Angela Maas is the managing editor of* Employee Benefit News, *a monthly magazine that provides information on group insurance, health care, and life and disability insurance.*

Health care fraud is one of the most prevalent and troubling crimes in the United States today. Authorities estimate that over $100 million per day is lost to health care fraud, which overtaxes insurance companies and consequently raises health insurance premiums for consumers. Health care fraud takes many forms, including phantom billing, where providers charge for services never performed; upcoding, where insurers are billed for more expensive services than were provided; and the performance of unnecessary medical procedures. Although Congress has passed a number of laws to combat health care fraud, experts believe that it will take consumers, insurance companies, and the government working together to solve the problem.

A cardiologist performs a number of unnecessary open-heart surgeries. A pharmacist dilutes a cancer drug that is prescribed to thousands of patients. A small business owner can't afford to provide medical insurance for his employees, so he has his own insurance extended to them by listing them all as his dependents.

All of these instances illustrate one of the most prevalent, and most costly, crimes today: health care fraud.

Statistics from the Center for Medicare and Medicaid Services show that Americans spent more than $1.7 trillion on health care in 2003. Combined with the fact that industry experts estimate that anywhere from 3% to 10% of this total is lost to health care fraud, that would put the minimum amount spent on health care fraud at over $100 million—per day.

"If that doesn't get people's attention, we're in trouble," says Michael Costello, director of investigation support for the Washington, D.C.–based National Health Care Anti-Fraud Association, founded in 1985 by several private health insurers and federal/state law enforcement officials.

Although fraud certainly isn't new to the health care industry, these crimes and efforts to stop them have been steadily receiving more attention. And although many insurance companies and government offices have been addressing fraud for more than a decade, most consumers didn't have much knowledge of the problem until the higher premiums and copays of the last five years or so began prompting questions about health care costs. Many experts feel that it will be the combination of consumers' vigilance and the insurance carriers' and the government's efforts that will make the difference in the battle to stop health care fraud and to reduce the various costs associated with it.

## Types of Fraud

Health care fraud can take many different forms, which is much of the reason why it's so difficult to detect. Providers, such as doctors, hospitals or physical therapists, as well as consumers can engage in fraud, and crimes may be committed by singular individuals or wide-reaching rings of people.

Common fraudulent provider practices are charging for services never performed (phantom billing), misrepresenting services (performing a tummy tuck and billing it to an insurance company as a hernia operation or an appendectomy, for example), upcoding (billing for a more expensive service than the one provided) and performing unnecessary medical procedures (such as paying patients cash, food or cigarettes in order to operate on them and then billing the insurance company for the service).

Furthermore, the BlueCross BlueShield Association reports that pharmaceutical fraud, in its various forms, is on the rise. A rash of impersonators masquerading as health professionals in order to acquire patients' insurance information has also been recently seen. Even the sharing of health insurance cards and adding non-family members to a policy are types of schemes. The plots are diverse and always changing, allowing people to stay one step ahead of the authorities.

"Most providers get into health care for the right reasons," says Joel Portice, vice president of healthcare solutions for Fair Isaac, a Minneapolis-based global provider of analytics and decision technology, "but there is enough opportunity when you have five billion claims in the system to change something, to add a procedure to the bill. The opportunities are there."

## Deeper Issues

Consumers need only to look at their health insurance premiums and copayments to recognize the impact of health care fraud. Each year the cost of health care has increased, and with it, fraud.

Costello points out that in 2000, 13.3% of the GDP was consumed with health care costs; in 2002, it was 14.9%. In 2010, projections put that number at 17%, and at 18.4% for 2013. "Our economy is not growing that fast," says Costello. "It can't keep up."

"When the cost of health insurance increases, it robs employers' abilities to pay their employees' benefits and salaries," says Byron Hollis, the national anti-fraud director of the Blue-Cross BlueShield Association, based in Washington, D.C. "It steals from the business directly by increasing employee health care costs and negatively impacting the bottom line in the same way other forms of theft would. In order to stay competitive, a business must raise the price of its goods or services, or decrease what it pays employees both in salaries and benefits."

> *All of the experts agree that it will take companies and consumers working together to combat the health care fraud problem.*

A company's reputation is also impacted, says Jose Tabuena, manager with global service provider KPMG LLP's Forensic Services, based in Dallas: "Whether it is a fraud that the company committed or the company is a victim, it hurts either way." Morale issues arise in either situation; employees may question whether they are working with a quality organization, which could in turn impact turnover and retention. The question of how vulnerable a company is also occurs.

## Patients Could Be Harmed

Patient harm is an additional problem. With an increase in unnecessary surgeries and procedures, this is becoming a real issue. For example, one "rent-a-patient" scheme involved about 100 clinics in California that recruited thousands of patients to travel to California and undergo outpatient surgery. The people were paid hundreds of dollars in cash, and then insurance companies were billed for tens and hundreds of thousands of dollars. Diluting medication, improperly prescribing medication and billing for but withholding treatment are also common risks.

Many consumers are unaware that most health insurance carriers have lifetime caps, and "false reporting can use up what is available to the patient," says Costello. He also points out that false reports will become part of a patient's record, meaning that a false illness would be a pre-existing condition that may not be covered by a different insurer later should it be an actual problem.

## Anti-Fraud Efforts

Insurers are fighting back against fraud with a diverse array of solutions. Many insurance companies have started their own investigation units, as have many corporations; those without in-house fraud experts will often outsource the position. For example, CIGNA started a special investigations team more than 20 years ago; [in 2003], their unit saved the company and its customers more than $65 million in unpaid, fraudulent claims, says Ken Faustine, a director in the special investigations unit, which is based in Hartford, Conn. In fact, most states have some sort of regulations that require special investigation units, anti-fraud plans or a combination of both. Companies are also investing in fraud detection software solutions, which analyze claims and try to detect and anticipate patterns.

The FBI established its Health Care Fraud Unit in 1992 as a separate unit within the Financial Crimes Section of the Criminal Investigative Division. The unit actually classified health care fraud as the No. 1 white-collar crime for many years until corporate fraud overtook it in 2002, knocking it down to its current

No. 2 position. It is actively investigating about 2,400 cases, as investigators work with private insurers, Medicaid, Medicare, and various other federal and state agencies, such as the Department of Health and Human Services Office of Inspector General. They tend to focus their efforts on criminal cases with national impact, such as organized criminal groups and health care chains.

> **Some worry that anti-fraud efforts may result in decreased quality of patient care.**

The National Health Care Anti-Fraud Association [NHCAA], which boasts about 20 members in the public sector and about 100 from the private, has two goals: first, to facilitate the exchange of information necessary to conduct criminal health care fraud investigations and second, to train investigators in the field on how to look for fraud as well as how to investigate it once they suspect it exists.

"We stay abreast of evolving schemes and adjust to trends we see," says the NHCAA's Costello. "We feel we are on top of the fraud picture because we are in daily contact with insurance companies and agencies."

## Anti-Fraud Laws

A number of laws dealing with health care fraud have been passed, most notably the Health Insurance Portability and Accountability Act in 1996. HIPAA provides funding for anti-fraud activities, including coordinating federal, state and local anti-fraud efforts, conducting investigations, providing guidance to the health care industry and establishing a national data bank containing final actions against health care providers. While establishing health care fraud as a federal criminal offense, the law provides for a federal prison term of up to 10 years for the basic crime; if the fraud results in the injury of a patient, the term can double to 20 years, and if a patient dies, the sentence can be life in federal prison.

But all of the experts agree that it will take companies and consumers working together to combat the health care fraud problem.

"Becoming alert to health care fraud requires no lifestyle

changes or complicated details," says the BlueCross BlueShield Association's Hollis. "By simply understanding what fraud looks like and taking a few simple steps to recognize and report it, the potential for savings is dramatic—approaching $85 billion a year, according to industry reports."

Tim Delaney, chief of the FBI's health care fraud unit, agrees that consumer interest has led to a greater awareness of health care fraud, and thus an increase in costs saved and recovered. He cites hotlines and explanations of benefits on medical forms as two actions that have been beneficial to the efforts.

"Years ago people thought, I'm covered by insurance, I don't need to worry about anything,'" says Costello. "But with rising premiums and copays, consumers have begun paying more attention." "As consumers become more cognizant of fraud, this will reduce it as well," says Mohit Ghose, director of public affairs with Washington, D.C.–based America's Health Insurance Plans. "More transparency is key. Consumers will ask for this, as well as ask what they're getting for their money."

## More Potential Problems

However, combating fraud brings up a number of other troubling issues. Some worry that anti-fraud efforts may result in decreased quality of patient care; in 2000, the *Journal of the American Medical Association* indicated that nearly one out of three physicians said that it was necessary to defraud the health care system in order to supply high-quality medical care.

Others are concerned that the costs of anti-fraud efforts may have the potential of offsetting the savings from fraud prevention. Fair Isaac [business corporation's Joel] Portice says that it depends on the plan itself, but if this is actually the case, "it is not a good solution. It's up to the technology community to provide solutions that have positive returns."

While state regulations regarding health care fraud are enacted with the best intentions, some are also plagued by contradictions among the requirements, says Costello. Many states have statutes that require companies to pay insurance claims within 30 to 45 days. But when one of those states also mandates that companies doing business in that state must have a special investigation unit that investigates suspected health care fraud, an investigation during this small window of time is an impossibility.

"We cannot say that a company must pay a claim in this

time and also aggressively pursue fraud," says Costello.

Another problem, ironically enough, concerns HIPAA itself. When the law was written, the resources were scheduled to be capped and flatlined in 2003. All of the programs have been affected, forcing units like the FBI to have to cut resources. In 1999, the bureau had 500 agents working for the health care fraud unit across the country, an increase of 388 agents from 1992. In 2004, it had about 480 agents employed in this capacity. Delaney reports that they are seeking legislative action in response to the funding.

## Health Care Fraud Investigations Decrease

[The September 11, 2001, terrorist attacks have] also drawn much of the FBI's focus, leading to the number of active health care fraud investigations and convictions to decrease as well.

Some experts counter that these decreasing instances of investigations and convictions could also be seen as the positive results of anti-fraud efforts: The numbers of instances have decreased because they are catching more of the criminals, getting a better handle on schemes and anticipating criminals' next moves by becoming more educated in their modus operandi. And many numbers do support this point of view. The BlueCross BlueShield Association reports that its anti-fraud efforts resulted in savings and recoveries of $240 million in 2003, a 52% increase from the previous year.

And while other statistics may show only a slight increase, or even a decrease, in convictions from year to year, it is important to remember that health care fraud investigations and convictions take about two to three years on average, with many of the larger cases lasting twice that long and convicting fewer people but recouping much more significant amounts of money. For example, in the recent Columbia/HCA Healthcare Corp. case, while only a handful of people were actually convicted, the nation's largest hospital chain agreed to pay the government $745 million to settle allegations of billing fraud.

## What the Future Holds

No one believes that health care fraud is a problem that is going to be solved any time soon. Certainly inroads can be made, but most experts agree that the numbers will most likely continue to grow.

"I think the amount of fraud is fairly high," says Hollis. "I think we're getting only the tip of the iceberg."

While some agree with this, others are more hesitant. "The extent of this is impossible to gauge," says Costello. "We don't know how big the iceberg actually is."

"No one accurately knows how much fraud is out there and how much it costs," says Tabuena. "No one knows what they didn't find. It is hard to know what you're looking for, to try to keep up with new schemes. We can't measure what we haven't seen."

# 11

# Comprehensive Health Care Reform Is Unlikely

## Jonathan Oberlander

*Jonathan Oberlander is a political scientist and assistant professor of social medicine in the School of Medicine at the University of North Carolina, Chapel Hill. He is also the author of* The Political Life of Medicare, *and coauthor of* The Path to Universal Health Care.

After President Bill Clinton's efforts to enact universal health care in 1994 failed, many politicians realized that trying to revamp America's ailing health care system was politically dangerous. In consequence, political efforts toward comprehensive health care reform stalled. Instead, proponents of reform have looked to the private sector to effect change. Unfortunately, despite claims by advocates of managed care that this system satisfactorily keeps health care costs down, health care costs are rising. Recent reform efforts designed to regulate managed care plans and permit patients to sue HMOs are unlikely to solve America's health care problems. America needs a comprehensive approach to reform such as a national health insurance policy.

The US health care system is often erroneously labelled a private health care system. In fact, the United States has a mixed system of public and private insurance, though the word "system" connotes much more organization and logic than is actually at work. Most working-age Americans receive health insurance through their employers. Medicare, a federal government program similar in structure to Canada's single-payer medicare insurance, provides health insurance to all Americans over 65 years of age as well as to persons with disabilities or end-stage renal disease. Medicaid, a jointly funded federal-state program, covers low-income Americans (it reaches about 40% of the poor), including seniors who "spend down" their incomes and assets to a level that qualifies them for Medicaid-funded nursing-home care. In between those covered by this hodgepodge of private and public plans, however, lies a substantial population without any health insurance at all.

## America's Uninsured

In 2000, 14% of Americans lacked health insurance. About 80% of the uninsured are either workers or live in families with workers. They typically have low-wage jobs or work in small businesses in which the employer does not offer health insurance or, if it is offered, they cannot afford to purchase it. The uninsured are disproportionately of low income. In 2000, one-third of the poor were uninsured, and two-thirds of uninsured adults had incomes less than 200% of the federal poverty line, or US$26,580 (Can$39,498) for a family of 3. Substantially more black (18.5%) and Hispanic (32%) than white (13%) Americans were uninsured in 2000.

Many Americans mistakenly believe that the uninsured obtain adequate care from hospital emergency rooms and other charity sources. Studies have consistently found, however, that the uninsured receive significantly less medical care than the insured. Nearly 25% of uninsured children and 40% of uninsured adults have no regular source of medical care. The uninsured are much more likely to delay or forgo needed treatment, have their conditions diagnosed at a later stage and be admitted to hospital for avoidable conditions. Moreover, inadequate insurance coverage carries with it financial as well as medical risks: the costs of medical treatment are a leading cause of bankruptcy in the United States. Indeed, about half of all bankruptcies in the United States "involve a medical reason or large medical debt."

## Favourable Circumstances but No Improvement

The number of uninsured individuals actually declined from 1998 to 1999, from 44.3 to 42.6 million, and in 2000 fell again to 38.7 million (though this latter drop was mainly due to statistical adjustments in how the government counts the uninsured). Yet perhaps most striking is not the decrease but, rather, that it took so long to happen and that the overall trend in the past decade remained one of an expanding uninsured population. Since the early 1990s, the United States has enjoyed ideal conditions for an expansion of health insurance. The economy has gone through an unprecedented era of sustained growth, the rates of general inflation and unemployment have remained low, and the rate of health care inflation has moderated. Still, from 1990 to 1998 the number of uninsured people increased by nearly 10 million.

> *About half of all bankruptcies in the United States 'involve a medical reason or large medical debt.'*

That even these favourable circumstances did not generate any significant expansion of health insurance is disquieting. And future trends are no more encouraging. The US economy slowed in 2000, and the unemployment rate rose. This economic downturn generated new ranks of the uninsured: the recent decline in the uninsured rate has ended. Because most Americans receive health insurance through their employer, a recession would have a strong negative impact on access to insurance. For the foreseeable future, then, the number of uninsured Americans is likely to continue to grow.

## The Politics of Health Reform

National health insurance periodically emerged on the US political agenda during the 20th century and was often tantalizingly close to enactment. The most recent failure came in 1994, with the defeat of the Health Security Act, sponsored by President Bill Clinton (and drafted under the guidance of his wife, Hillary). Clinton proposed to achieve universal coverage in the United States by mandating that all employers provide private health insurance to their employees and by giving small businesses and unemployed Americans subsidies with which to purchase insurance. However, the Clinton plan triggered fierce opposition from the insurance industry (which disliked the proposed regulation of behaviours, such as experience rating, which has enabled them to charge higher premiums for sick patients), the business community (which criticized the employer mandate), ideologic conservatives (who saw the plan as an unwarranted nationalization of the health care system) and large segments of the public (who were anxious about the plan's emphasis on moving patients into HMOs). Confronted with this opposition and the lack of a liberal political majority in Congress, the act was defeated. The American Medical Association, which initially endorsed and then waffled on the idea of universal insurance coverage, did not play a prominent role in the 1993/94 debate, a sign of its deteriorating influence on US health politics.

One legacy of the Clinton plan's failure has been caution regarding health policy. Many politicians took the lesson of the plan's demise to be that comprehensive reform—transforming the US system into one of national health insurance, like Canadian medicare—is not politically feasible. Consequently, talk of attaining universal coverage has all but disappeared. Neither of the 2 major parties' presidential candidates in the 2000 election, Al Gore and George W. Bush, offered plans for universal insurance coverage. None of the plans currently under serious consideration in Congress attempts to cover all of the uninsured [as of July 2002]. And even one of the few organized advocates for the uninsured, the consumer group Families USA, has toned down its calls for universal coverage in favour of more modest policy goals.

## Absence of Proposals for Universal Coverage

What is remarkable about the absence of proposals for universal coverage in the period 1999–2001 is that the fiscal circumstances of the United States appeared to be conducive to their adoption. After 2 decades of budget deficits, the federal government in 2000 ran a sizeable budget surplus, projected at $5.6 trillion over the next decade. It has long been assumed that the lack of affordability of a public program was a central barrier, particularly in an era of sizeable federal deficits in which large spending initiatives were politically constrained and tax increases taboo. Now, though, the affordability argument has been exposed as a fallacy. Despite the availability of a budget surplus that could be used to pay the costs of covering the uninsured, universal coverage did not emerge as a central political issue in 2000/01. Instead, political attention focused on improving the medical experiences of the already insured through regulation of managed care and expansion of Medicare to cover outpatient prescription drugs.

> *Universal coverage remains an elusive reform in the United States, and the uninsured continue to live in an 'aura of invisibility.'*

It is clear that the most relevant fact about US health politics is not that some 15% of the population are uninsured but that about 85% of the population are insured. Those who are insured are generally satisfied with their own medical care, even if they think poorly of the system as a whole; consequently, they are not a strong constituency for change. Indeed, any reform that threatens to alter the medical care arrangements of the insured is likely to provoke public opposition. The formidable constituency against reform is mobilized, wealthy and politically influential. Meanwhile, the uninsured are disproportionately low-income, unorganized and apparently politically expendable. As the Clinton plan exemplified, the political benefits to a president and legislators willing to take on a trillion-dollar health care industry that opposes reform are uncertain, but the costs are certain to be high. The result is that universal coverage remains an elusive reform in the United States, and the uninsured continue to live in an "aura of invisibility."

## Expanding Incremental Reforms

Although there is currently little appetite for comprehensive reforms that would assure universal coverage, there is momentum for incremental measures that would reduce the ranks of the uninsured. Two main pathways to improved coverage have emerged. The first approach is to expand existing public insurance programs, including Medicaid, which provides insurance to about 40% of the poor, and the State Children's Health Insurance Program (SCHIP), which provides insurance to children living in families with incomes up to 200% of the federal poverty line. Proponents of this approach would change eligibility requirements for these programs, opening them up to more of the poor and near-poor (e.g., to parents of children enrolled in SCHIP). One of the more ambitious plans would extend Medicaid and SCHIP coverage, without premiums or cost-sharing, to all persons with incomes below 150% of the federal poverty line and subsidize enrolment for persons with incomes up to 300%. It is estimated that this plan would extend eligibility for public insurance to over 25 million Americans who are currently uninsured. Most plans, however, would not expand coverage so broadly and would thus not reach most of the uninsured.

## Problems with Tax Credits

A second approach—one favoured by the Bush administration—is to adopt tax credits that would help the uninsured purchase private insurance. This approach appears to be especially attractive given the political appeal of tax cuts and the promise of expanded coverage with minimal government involvement. Most tax-credit proposals would target individuals, though some plans have instead focused on credits for employers. Credits could be refundable, so that even low-income persons who do not pay federal income tax would be eligible.

There are several problems, however, with tax-credit proposals in particular and incremental reforms more generally. The main problem with tax credits is the mismatch between the size of the credits that are being proposed and the cost of insurance. The average annual premium of a health insurance policy in the United States is now more than US$6000 (Can$8910) for a family and more than $3000 for an individual. President Bush's proposal would provide a tax credit of only $2000 to a family and $1000 to an individual. It is questionable how much difference these tax credits would make to the uninsured, many of whom have little disposable income. This is especially true because insurance for individuals has much higher administrative costs than group insurance, and consequently higher premiums.

More fundamentally, neither tax credits nor expanded public insurance does anything to control medical care spending. The debate has changed markedly since the early 1990s, when concerns over rapidly rising costs and the economic competitiveness of US firms drove health reform. Politically, the absence of cost containment in the current proposals is hardly surprising. After all, health care costs equal the total incomes of the providers of medical care, a group comprising not merely physicians but also insurers, hospitals, nursing homes, pharmaceutical companies and all those selling medical services and products. Any attempt to restrain national health spending is viewed by providers as an assault on their livelihood, which triggers intense opposition. An understandable reading by US politicians of the Clinton reform debacle is that expanding coverage is difficult; simultaneously mandating spending controls would be political suicide.

> *Any attempt to restrain national health spending is viewed by providers as an assault on their livelihood, which triggers intense opposition.*

Yet there are signs that the moderate medical care inflation that made inattention to cost control comfortable is ending. Absent cost control, then, incremental reforms may become self-defeating, with high rates of medical care inflation leading to higher-than-expected program costs, which could make expansion of insurance coverage less affordable and politically problematic.

## How Managed Care Works

US medical care has long been the most expensive in the world. The defeat of comprehensive health reform in 1994 did not obviate the pressures to control health spending; rather, it shifted the engine of control to the private sector. Employers looking to hold down their medical bills embraced managed care and, in a staggeringly short time, managed care became the norm. By 2000, 92% of persons with employer-sponsored insurance were enrolled in a managed care plan. Managed care has also spread to public programs for the elderly, poor and disabled—Medicare and Medicaid—though enrolment in such plans is generally lower than for the employer-sponsored population.

Managed care has come to refer to a wide range of health plans and practices that depart from the traditional US model of insurance. In the traditional model, insured patients chose their physician; physicians treated patients with absolute clinical autonomy; insurers generally paid physicians whatever they billed on a fee-for-service basis; and employers paid premiums for their workers to private insurers, footing the bill regardless of its cost. Managed care has altered all of these arrangements. As a consequence of not having national health insurance, cost control in the United States has focused more on setting limits on the individual medical encounter ("managing care") than on establishing budgetary limits for the entire health care sector.

## Major Changes with Managed Care

The rise of managed care has brought about 4 major changes in US medical care. First is the substantial decline in traditional indemnity-insurance arrangements, which allowed unfettered access to physicians and unregulated delivery of medical care. The proportion of Americans with employer-sponsored indemnity coverage declined from 95% in 1978 to 14% by 1998. This drop was accompanied by an increase in enrolment in a wide variety of managed-care insurance programs, including HMOs, Preferred Provider Organizations (PPOs) and Point of Service plans (POSs). Not only did HMOs grow in enrolment—from 36.5 million in 1990 to 58.2 million in 1995—but they also changed substantially in form. In particular, there has been rapid growth in for-profit HMOs as well as network and individual-practice association models that contract with providers; in contrast, group or staff-model HMOs (such as Kaiser Permanente) own their facilities, and their physicians work exclusively for them. Yet, while they continue to be regarded as the symbol of managed care, the growth of HMOs has stalled in recent years, and more Americans with job-provided insurance are now enrolled in PPOs (41%) than in HMOs (29%).

> *US physicians probably experience more intrusion into their clinical lives than physicians anywhere in the industrialized world.*

Second, patients in managed care receive full coverage for services only if they choose a physician within the plan's network. In the case of HMOs, patients receive no coverage if they see an out-of-network provider. In some plans, patients must go through a gatekeeper, typically a primary care physician, to obtain a specialty referral. The corollary is that most insurers no longer contract with all physicians in a community. Rather, they contract with a limited number of doctors, negotiating price discounts in exchange for guaranteed patient volume and excluding high-cost providers.

## How Insurers Control Physicians

Third, physicians' clinical decisions are now regularly subject to external review by insurance plans. Indeed, US physicians probably experience more intrusion into their clinical lives than physicians anywhere in the industrialized world, an ironic development given that the American Medical Association long opposed national health insurance as a threat to clinical autonomy. Under utilization-review arrangements, physicians may have to seek permission from the patient's insurance company for admission to hospital, diagnostic tests or medical procedures. Utilization review and physician profiling may also occur after treatment, with the goal of identifying "inappropriate" or "excessive" care according to the insurer's standards. Proponents of managed care argue that these practices can not only control costs but also enhance quality of care—for instance, by assuring adherence to evidence-based medicine.

Fourth, insurers no longer give physicians a blank cheque; instead, they may dictate not only the price of reimbursement but also the form. This has led to the widespread adoption of predetermined fee schedules for physician payment by managed care plans, which seek discounts from "normal" fees. HMOs have also adopted capitated payment, often focusing on primary care providers. Under capitated payment, physicians receive a set amount for each patient enrolled in their practice, regardless of that patient's actual use of services. The stated aim is to avoid the financial incentive for overtreatment inherent in fee-for-service payment. Another important change in payment arrangements is the introduction of bonuses and other incentives for physicians to meet targets in providing care. Frequently these incentives are aimed at ensuring that physicians hold down costs in a capitated environment; for instance, bonuses may be provided to physicians whose rate of admission to hospital for their patient pool is lower than the insurer's target. Along with capitation, these arrangements put the incomes of many physicians at substantial risk.

# The Impact of Management Care on Costs and Quality

Since the advent of managed care in the early 1990s, health care spending in the United States has slowed. From 1993 to 1998, the share of gross domestic product (GDP) devoted to national health expenditures declined from 13.7% to 13.5%, and premiums for employer-sponsored health insurance actually grew more slowly than the per capita GDP. However, the United States continues to spend far more on medical care than any other nation: in 1998, it spent $4270 per capita, compared with $2400 in Germany, which spent the second-highest amount, and $2250 in Canada.

There is substantial disagreement among analysts about the significance of the relative success of the United States in controlling health care spending during the mid-1990s. Some observers believe that this experience demonstrates managed care's effectiveness in controlling costs and the efficiencies inherent in strategies such as selective contracting, utilization review and capitation. Others attribute the slowdown to a one-time switch from indemnity insurance that cannot be duplicated or to temporary circumstances that cannot be sustained, such as marketing strategies that led insurers to underprice their products to expand market share. The long-term cost-containment potential of managed care consequently remains uncertain. However, health care spending in 1999 and 2000 rose at higher rates: insurance premiums increased by 8.3% in 2000, and even larger increases were expected for 2001. This suggests that the era of low medical care inflation is over and that managed care's ability to restrain spending has been exaggerated.

Evidence for the impact of managed care on the quality of care is mixed. Most studies have found little difference in quality of care between traditional insurers and managed care plans, though there is evidence of worse outcomes for chronically ill seniors in HMOs. That quality of care in many cases did not deteriorate despite reduced volume and intensity of services suggests that the previous standard of "unmanaged" care incorporated significant amounts of unnecessary services. However, these findings also cast doubt on the premise that managed care is improving quality through practice guidelines, preventive care, primary care, disease management, integrated delivery systems and other strategies. Too often, these strategies exist more as marketing labels than as workable or proven innovations, though that has not stopped them from being aggressively promoted outside the United States, often to receptive audiences looking for new levers to control costs and improve quality and consumer service. Yet, so far, managed care plans have not consistently implemented these practices, and market competition has not resulted in significant quality improvements. Instead, plans have focused on managing costs, a decision reinforced by employers, who are much more likely to select insurance on the basis of price than on the basis of quality.

## The Managed Care Backlash

Regardless of the evidence, there is strong sentiment among both physicians and patients that managed care is harming quality of care. Consequently, there has been a push to enact patients' bills of rights and other laws that regulate the behaviour of managed care plans. Virtually all of the 50 US states now have such laws on the books, and Congress is debating federal legislation that would permit patients to sue HMOs,[1] guarantee access to specialists and establish procedures for appealing health plan decisions denying coverage or medical care. If adopted, this legislation will no doubt provide political benefits to its sponsors, who can assure the voting public that they are doing something about HMO abuses. Its impact on patients and quality of care is less certain. The legislation is sufficiently vague that it is difficult to know how strictly it will be implemented and how much it will change health plan behaviour. Moreover, the proposed law does not address issues such as financial bonuses for physicians and the incentives of capitation that significantly affect patient care.

## No Closer to Solving Problems

After a decade of change, the United States appears to be no closer to solving the problems of cost control and access that have characterized its health care system for the past 3 decades. The question is, after the political system takes care of the al-

1. In 2001 a "patients' bill of rights," which, among other things, would allow patients to sue HMOs, was introduced into Congress. The bill did not pass either house. However, in 2004, after a Supreme Court ruling denying patients the right to sue HMOs for damages caused by their refusal to pay for needed treatment, a new patients' bill of rights was introduced into Congress. The bill was still pending as this volume went to press.

ready insured through managed-care protections and expanded Medicare benefits for the elderly, what will it do for the uninsured?

The September 11, 2001, bombings of the World Trade Center and the Pentagon have triggered a new period in US politics, dominated in the short term by President Bush's war on terrorism. In the aftermath of the terrorist strikes, "United we stand" became a national slogan of solidarity. Some health reformers hope that this communitarian spirit and the renewed faith of Americans in government will give national health insurance a new life. And enactment of incremental expansions of public insurance programs and tax credits for the uninsured is a real possibility. But it is not clear that health reform will move beyond these limited steps, which would leave the bulk of the uninsured population untouched. Absent a sustained economic downturn that makes the middle class anxious about their own coverage, prospects for universal coverage and comprehensive health care reform remain dim. The more things change in US health care policy, the more they seem to stay the same.

# Organizations to Contact

The editors have compiled the following list of organizations concerned with the issues debated in this book. The descriptions are derived from materials provided by the organizations. All have publications or information available for interested readers. The list was compiled on the date of publication of the present volume; names, addresses, phone and fax numbers, and e-mail addresses may change. Be aware that many organizations take several weeks or longer to respond to inquiries, so allow as much time as possible.

**Alliance for Advancing Nonprofit Healthcare**
PO Box 41015, Washington, DC 20018
(877) 299-6497
Web site: www.nonprofithealthcare.org

The Alliance for Advancing Nonprofit Healthcare seeks to enable the abilities of nonprofit health care organizations to serve society and their individual communities. It provides a voice for nonprofit health care organizations through advocacy, public education, and research. Some of its publications include *Costs, Commitment, and Locality: A Comparison of for-Profit and Not-for-Profit Health Plans, Advancing the Role of Nonprofit Health Care,* and *Nonprofit Health Insurers: The Financial Story Wall Street Doesn't Tell.*

**American Council on Science and Health (ACSH)**
1995 Broadway, 2nd Fl., New York, NY 10023-5860
(212) 362-7044 • fax: (212) 362-4919
e-mail: whelan@acsh.org • Web site: www.acsh.org

ACSH provides consumers with scientifically balanced evaluations of food, chemicals, the environment, and human health. It publishes the quarterly magazine *Priorities for Health,* the semiannual *News from ACSH,* and the book *Issues in Nutrition.*

**American Enterprise Institute (AEI)**
1150 Seventeenth St. NW, Washington, DC 20036
(202) 862-5800 • fax: (202) 862-7178
Web site: www.aei.org

The American Interprise Institute for Public Policy Research is dedicated to preserving and strengthening the foundations of freedom—limited government, private enterprise, vital cultural and political institutions, and a strong foreign policy and national defense—through scholarly research, open debate, and publications. Founded in 1943, AEI researches economics and trade; social welfare and health; government tax, spending, regulatory, and legal policies; U.S. politics; international affairs; and U.S. defense and foreign policies. The institute publishes dozens of books and hundreds of article and reports each year and a policy magazine, the *American Enterprise.*

### American Medical Association (AMA)
515 N. State St., Chicago, IL 60610
(312) 464-4818 • fax: (312) 464-4184
Web site: www.ama-assn.org

The AMA is the primary professional association of physicians in the United States. Founded in 1847, it disseminates information to its members and the public concerning medical breakthroughs, medical and health legislation, educational standards for physicians, and other issues concerning medicine and health care. The AMA operates a library and offers many publications, including the weekly *JAMA: The Journal of the American Medical Association*, the weekly newspaper *American Medical News*, and journals covering specific medical specialties.

### American Public Health Association (APHA)
800 I St. NW, Washington, DC 20001-3710
(202) 777-2742 • fax: (202) 777-2534 • TTY: (202) 777-2500
e-mail: comments@apha.org • Web site: www.apha.org

Founded in 1872, the American Public Health Association consists of more than fifty thousand individuals and organizations that support health promotion. Its members represent more than fifty public health occupations, including researchers, practitioners, administrators, teachers, and other health care workers. Some of APHA's publications include the *American Journal of Public Health* and a monthly newspaper, the *Nation's Health*.

### American Public Human Services Association (APHSA)
810 First St. NE, Suite 500, Washington, DC 20002
(202) 682-0100 • fax: (202) 289-6555
e-mail: jpatterson@aphsa.org • Web site: www.aphsa.org

APHSA is an organization of members of human services agencies and other individuals interested in human service issues. The association's mission is to develop, promote, and implement public human services policies that improve the health and well-being of families, children, and adults. It's publications include the professional journal *Policy & Practice* and the annual *Public Human Services Directory.*

### American Society of Law, Medicine, and Ethics (ASLME)
765 Commonwealth Ave., Suite 1634, Boston, MA 02215
(617) 262-4990 • fax: (617) 437-7596
e-mail: info@aslme.org • Web site: www.aslme.org

The mission of ASLME is to provide high-quality scholarship, debate, and critical thought to professionals in the fields of law, health care, policy, and ethics. The society acts as a source of guidance and information through the publication of two quarterlies, the *Journal of Law, Medicine & Ethics* and the *American Journal of Law & Medicine*. More information about ASLME is available on its Web site.

**Brookings Institution**
775 Massachusetts Ave. NW, Washington, DC 20036-2188
(202) 797-6000 • fax: (202) 797-6004
Web site: www.brook.edu

Founded in 1927, the institution is a liberal research and education organization that publishes material on economics, government, and foreign policy. It strives to serve as a bridge between scholarship and public policy, bringing new knowledge to the attention of decision makers and providing scholars with improved insight into public policy issues. The Brookings Institution produces hundreds of abstracts and reports on health care with topics ranging from Medicaid to persons with disabilities.

**Cato Institute**
1000 Massachusetts Ave. NW, Washington, DC 20001-5403
(202) 842-0200 • fax: (202) 842-3490
e-mail: cato@cato.org • Web site: www.cato.org

The Cato Institute is a libertarian public policy research foundation dedicated to limiting the role of government and protecting individual liberties. Its Health and Welfare Studies Department works to formulate and popularize a free-market agenda for health care reform. The institute publishes the quarterly magazine *Regulation*, the bimonthly *Cato Policy Report*, and numerous books and commentaries, hundreds of which relate to health care.

**Center for Studying Health System Change (HSC)**
600 Maryland Ave. SW, #550, Washington, DC 20024
(202) 484-5261 • fax: (202) 484-9258
e-mail: hscinfo@hschange.org • Web site: www.hschange.org

The Center for Studying Health System Change is a nonpartisan policy research organization. HSC designs and conducts studies focused on the U.S. health care system to inform the thinking and decisions of policy makers in government and private industry. In addition, HSC studies contribute more broadly to the body of health care policy research that enables decision makers to understand change and the national and local market forces driving that change. HSC publishes issue briefs, community reports, tracking reports, data bulletins, and journal articles based on its research.

**Consumers Union**
101 Truman Ave., Yonkers, NY 10703-1057
(914) 378-2000
Web site: www.consumersunion.org

Consumers Union, publisher of *Consumer Reports*, is an independent, nonprofit testing and information organization serving only consumers. It is a comprehensive source for unbiased advice about products and services, personal finance, health, health care, nutrition, and other consumer concerns. Since 1936 it has been testing products, informing the public, and protecting consumers.

**Healthcare Leadership Council (HLC)**
1001 Pennsylvania Ave. NW, Suite 550 South, Washington, DC 20004
(202) 452-8700 • fax: (202) 296-9561
Web site: www.hlc.org

The council is a forum in which health care industry leaders can jointly develop policies, plans, and programs that support a market-based health care system. HLC believes that America's health care system should value innovation and provide affordable, high-quality health care free from excessive government regulations. It offers the latest press releases on health issues and several public policy papers with titles such as "Empowering Consumers and Patients" and "Ensuring Responsible Government."

### Heritage Foundation
214 Massachusetts Ave. NE, Washington, DC 20002-4999
(800) 544-4843 • (202) 546-4400 • fax: (202) 546-8328
e-mail: pubs@heritage.org • Web site: www.heritage.org

The Heritage Foundation is a public policy research institute that advocates limited government and the free-market system. It believes that the private sector, not government, should be relied on to ease social problems. The Heritage Foundation publishes the quarterly *Policy Review*, as well as hundreds of monographs, background papers, and books.

### Institute for Health Freedom (IHF)
1825 Eye St. NW, Suite 400, Washington, DC 20006
(202) 429-6610 • fax: (202) 861-1973
e-mail: feedback@forhealthfreedom.org
Web site: www.forhealthfreedom.org

IHF is a nonpartisan, nonprofit research center established to bring the issues of personal freedom in choosing health care to the forefront of America's health policy debate. Its mission is to present the ethical and economic case for strengthening personal health freedom. IHF's research and analyses are published as policy briefings on subjects such as children's health care, monopoly in medicine, and legal issues. All are available on its Web site.

### Kaiser Family Foundation
2400 Sand Hill Rd., Menlo Park, CA 94025
(650) 854-9400 • (650) 854-4800
Web site: www.kff.org

The Henry J. Kaiser Family Foundation is an independent philanthropy focusing on the major health care issues facing the nation. The foundation is an independent voice and source of facts and analysis for policy makers, the media, the health care community, and the general public. It is primarily an operating organization that develops and runs its own research and communications programs, often in partnership with outside organizations. Foundation work is focused in three main areas: health policy, media and public education, and health and development in South Africa. The foundation publishes hundreds of papers, articles, and reports each year. Most are available on its Web site.

### National Center for Policy Analysis (NCPA)
601 Pennsylvania Ave. NW, Suite 900
South Building, Washington, DC 20004
(202) 628-6671 • fax: (202) 628-6474
e-mail: ncpa@public-policy.org • Web site: www.ncpa.org

NCPA is a nonprofit public policy research institute. It publishes the bi-monthly newsletter *Executive Alert* as well as numerous health care policy studies with titles such as "Saving Medicare" and "Medical Savings Accounts: Obstacles to Their Growth and Ways to Improve Them." Its Web site includes an extensive section on health care issues.

### National Coalition on Health Care
1200 G St. NW, Suite 750, Washington, DC 20005
(202) 638-7151 • fax: (202) 638-7166
e-mail: jthompson@nchc.org • Web site: www.nchc.org

The National Coalition on Health Care is a nonprofit, nonpartisan group that represents the nation's largest alliance working to improve America's health care and make it more affordable. The coalition offers several policy studies with titles ranging from "Why the Quality of U.S. Health Care Must Be Improved" to "The Rising Number of Uninsured Workers: An Approaching Crisis in Health Care Financing."

### National Institutes of Health (NIH)
9000 Rockville Pike, Bethesda, MD 20892
(301) 496-4000
e-mail: nihinfo@od.nih.gov • Web site: www.nih.gov

The NIH is made up of twenty-seven separate components, including the National Human Genome Research Institute and the National Cancer Institute. Its mission is to discover new knowledge that will improve everyone's health. In order to achieve this mission, the NIH conducts and supports research, helps train research investigators, and fosters the communication of medical information. The NIH also publishes online fact sheets, brochures, and handbooks.

### Physicians for a National Health Program (PNHP)
29 E. Madison St., Suite 602, Chicago, IL 60602
(312) 782-6006 • fax: (312) 782-6007
e-mail: pnhp@aol.com • Web site: www.pnhp.org

PNHP is a not-for-profit organization of physicians, medical students, and other health care professionals that supports a national health insurance program. Members of PNHP specifically believe that a single-payer system (in which the government finances health care but keeps the delivery of health care in mostly private hands) is the only solution to the United States' many health care problems. Its publications include *Physicians Proposal for Single-Payer National Health Insurance 2003* and *A National Long-Term Care Program for the United States.*

### Reason Foundation
3415 S. Sepulveda Blvd., Suite 400, Los Angeles, 90034
(310) 391-22454
Web site: www.reason.org

The Reason Foundation is a national research and education organization that explores and promotes public policy based on rationality and freedom. The Reason Foundation's public policy think tank—the Reason Public Policy Institute—promotes choice, competition, and a dynamic market economy as the foundation for human dignity and progress. The

Reason Foundation publishes the monthly *Reason Magazine* and the on-line *Reason Report* as well as many books including *Earth Report 2000*.

**Urban Institute**
2100 M St. NW, Washington, DC 20037
(202) 833-7200
e-mail: paffairs@ui.urban.org • Web site: www.urban.org

The Urban Institute investigates social and economic problems confronting the nation and analyzes efforts to solve these problems. In addition, it works to improve government decisions and to increase citizen awareness about important public choices. It offers a wide variety of resources, including books such as *Restructuring Medicare: Impacts on Beneficiaries* and *The Decline in Medical Spending Growth in 1996: Why Did It Happen?*

# Bibliography

## Books

Pat Armstrong and
Hugh Armstrong
*Universal Health Care: What the United States Can Learn from the Canadian Experience.* New York: New Press, 1999.

Donald Barlett and
James B. Steele
*Critical Condition: How Health Care in America Became Big Business and Bad Medicine.* New York: Doubleday, 2004.

Thomas S.
Bodenheimer and
Kevin Grumbach
*Understanding Health Policy.* Stamford, CT: McGraw-Hill/Appleton and Lange, 2001.

Jamie Court
*Making a Killing: HMOs and the Threat to Your Health.* Monroe, ME: Common Courage, 1999.

David M. Cutler
*Your Money or Your Life: Strong Medicine for America's Health Care System.* New York: Oxford University Press, 2004.

Norman Daniels,
Bruce Kennedy, and
Ichiro Kawachi
*Is Inequality Bad for Our Health?* Boston: Beacon, 2000.

Gerhard Falk
*Hippocrates Assailed.* Lanham, MD: University Press of America, 1999.

John P. Geyman
*Health Care in America: Can Our Ailing System Be Healed?* Boston: Buttersworth-Heinemann, 2001.

Newt Gingrich
*Saving Lives and Saving Money.* Arlington, VA: Alexis de Tocqueville Institution, 2003.

Colin Gordon
*Dead on Arrival: The Politics of Health Care in Twentieth-Century America.* Princeton, NJ: Princeton University Press, 2003.

George C. Halvorson
and George J. Isham
*Epidemic of Care: A Call for Safer, Better, and More Accountable Health Care.* San Francisco: Jossey-Bass, 2002.

Charlene Harrington
and Carroll L. Estes
*Health Policy: Crisis and Reform on the U.S. Health Care Delivery.* Boston: Jones and Bartlett, 2001.

Regina Herzlinger
*Market-Driven Healthcare: Who Wins, Who Loses in the Transformation of America's Largest Service Industry.* Cambridge, MA: Perseus, 1999.

David Himmelstein,
Steffie Woolhandler,
and Ida Hellander
*Bleeding the Patient: The Consequences of Corporate Health Care.* Monroe, ME: Common Courage, 2001.

| Institute for the Future | *Health and Health Care 2010: The Forecast, the Challenge.* San Francisco: Jossey-Bass, 2001. |
|---|---|
| J.D. Kleinke | *Oxymorons: The Myth of the U.S. Health Care System.* San Francisco: Jossey-Bass, 2001. |
| Richard D. Lamm | *The Brave New World of Health Care.* Golden, CO: Fulcrum, 2003. |
| Robert H. Lebow | *Health Care Meltdown.* Chambersburg, PA: Alan C. Hood, 2004. |
| Ein Lewin and Stuart Altman, eds. | *America's Health Care Safety Net: Intact but Endangered.* Washington, DC: National Academy, 2000. |
| Cynthia S. McCullough | *Creating Responsive Solutions to Healthcare Change.* Indianapolis, IN: Center Nursing, 2001. |
| Matthew Miller | *The 2% Solution.* New York: Public Affairs, 2003. |
| Ian Morrison | *Health Care in the New Millennium: Vision, Values, and Leadership.* San Francisco: Jossey-Bass, 2002. |
| Allyson M. Pollock | *The Privatisation of Our Health Care.* London: Verso, 2004. |
| Kevin Taft and Gillian Steward | *Clear Answers: The Economics and Politics of for-Profit Medicine.* Edmonton, Canada: University of Alberta Press, 2000. |
| Peter A. Weil, Richard J. Bogue, and Read L. Morton | *Achieving Success Through Community Leadership.* Chicago: Health Administration, 2001. |

## Periodicals

| Christa Altenstetter | "Insights from Health Care in Germany," *American Journal of Public Health*, January 2003. |
|---|---|
| Charles Babcock and Marianne Kolbasuk McGee | "Filter Out the Frauds," *Information Week*, June 28, 2004. |
| Gary Boulard | "Coverage Conundrum," *State Legislatures*, July/August 2004. |
| Dave Carpenter | "Insurers Reign," *Hospitals and Health Networks*, September 2003. |
| Kevin Clarke | "With Liberty and Health Care for All," *U.S. Catholic*, March 2004. |
| Jonathan Cohn | "Health Scare: The Next Big Health Care Crisis Is Now," *New Republic*, December 24, 2001. |
| Geoffrey Colvin | "What Do Voters Want? A Clean Bill of Health," *Fortune*, February 23, 2004. |
| *Congressional Digest* | "The Ongoing Medicare Debate," February 2004. |
| *Consumer Reports* | "The Unraveling of Health Insurance," July 2002. |

| Barbara Ehrenreich | "Gouging the Poor," *Progressive*, February 2004. |
| David Gergen | "The Elephant in the Room: Fixing the Healthcare System," *U.S. News & World Report*, December 9, 2002. |
| Chandrani Ghosh | "When Bean Counters Dispense Medicine," *Forbes*, April 29, 2002. |
| Howard Gleckman | "Who Should Get the Bill? Dispute over Health Insurance Reform," *Business Week*, March 4, 2002. |
| *Good Housekeeping* | "The Best HMO Story We've Heard," February 2002. |
| Scott Gottlieb | "Prevention Is Not a Cure: HMOs Abandon Prevention-Is-Cheaper Business Model," *American Spectator*, March/April 2002. |
| *Governing* | "Access Denied: Medical Costs for the Uninsured," February 2004. |
| Timothy Gower | "Blindsided," *Reader's Digest*, February 2004. |
| Brian Grow | "Health Insurance Scams Will Make You Sick," *Business Week*, August 19–26, 2002. |
| Devon M. Herrick | "Consumer Choice Is the Key to Health-Care Reform," *Consumers' Research*, November 2003. |
| Wil S. Hylton | "The View from Inside: Discussion of Sick on the Inside," Letters, *Harper's*, January 2004. |
| Brian R. Klepper, Patrick G. Hayes, and J. Brooks | "Saving American Health Care," *Journal of Ambulatory Care Management*, July 2002. |
| Penelope Lemov | "Healing Health Care," *Governing*, January 2004. |
| Donald W. Light | "Health Care for All: A Conservative Proposal," *Commonweal*, February 22, 2002. |
| Donald W. Light | "Universal Health Care: Lessons from the British Experience," *American Journal of Public Health*, January 2003. |
| W.W. McGuire | "The American Health System," *Vital Speeches of the Day*, March 15, 2002. |
| Haavi Morreim | "Let Contracts, Not 'Necessity' Guide the Health System: Deciding What Is Medically Necessary," *Consumers' Research*, December 2001. |
| John Nichols | "Healthy Debate," *Nation*, November 3, 2003. |
| Don Peck | "Putting a Value on Health," *Atlantic Monthly*, January/February 2004. |
| Kaja Perina | "Battling for Benefits," *Psychology Today*, March/April 2002. |
| Sally Pipes | "Is the Cure Worse than the Disease?" *Saturday Evening Post*, January/February 2004. |

| Tripp Quillman | "When Confidentiality Is Compromised: Confidentiality Breaches in Managed Care Mental Health Files," *Newsweek*, May 6, 2002. |
| Arnold S. Relman | "Restructuring the U.S. Health Care System," *Issues in Science and Technology*, Summer 2003. |
| Julius B. Richmond and Rashi Fein | "Health Insurance in the USA," *Science*, September 26, 2003. |
| Victor G. Rodwin | "The Health Care System Under French National Health Insurance: Lessons for Health Reform in the United States," *American Journal of Public Health*, January 2003. |
| Laurie Rubiner | "Insurance Required: Means of Achieving Universal Health Coverage," *Atlantic Monthly*, January/February 2004. |
| Michael Scherer | "Medicare's Hidden Bonanza," *Mother Jones*, March/April 2004. |
| Marc Siegel | "Coverage for No One," *Nation*, January 12–19, 2004. |
| Deborah A. Stone | "United States," *Journal of Health Politics, Policy and Law*, October 2000. |
| Rosemarie Sweeney | "Health Care Coverage for All," *American Family Physicians*, March 15, 2004. |
| Karen Tumulty | "Health Care Has a Relapse," *Time*, March 11, 2002. |

# Index